Indigenous Health Practices among the People of North East India

Indigenous Health Practices among the People of North East India

Sarthak Sengupta

KALPAZ

ISBN: 978-93-5128-243-3

First Published, 2018

Published by

Kalpaz Publications
C-30, Satyawati Nagar,
Delhi – 110052
E-mail: kalpaz@hotmail.com
Ph.: 9212142040

Printed at: G. Print Process, Delhi

Cataloging in Publication Data—DK

Courtesy: D.K. Agencies (P) Ltd. <docinfo@dkagencies.com>

Indigenous health practices among the people of North East India / [edited by] Sarthak Sengupta.
pages cm
Includes bibliographical references.
ISBN 9789351282433

1. Traditional medicine—India—Assam. 2. Traditional medicine—India, Northeastern. 3. Tribes—Health and hygiene—India—Assam. 4. Tribes—Health and hygiene—India, Northeastern. 5. Ethnobiology—India—Assam. 6. Ethnobiology—India, Northeastern. I. Sengupta, Sarthak, 1955- editor.

LCC R607.A87I53 2017 | DDC 610.954162 23

To

Late Professor Geeta Talukdar

for all of your affection and support towards
my research career

this one is in your honour

Contents

List of Tables

Preface

Indigenous knowledge cannot be verified by scientific criteria nor can science be agreeably assessed according to the doctrine of indigenous knowledge. Each is built on distinctive philosophies, methodologies, and criteria. Siegerist (1951) has stated that 'every culture had developed a system of medicine'. Anthropological studies of medicine as a social institution have shown that every human society has developed, according to premises implicit in its own culture, a system of values regarding health and diseases, as an also method of coping with them (Hasan, 1968). Indigenous medicine has sustained itself through processes deeply rooted in a society's socio-cultural complexes. Indigenous medicinal substances, their nature, axioms, and practices vary from one country to another, or more precisely, from one culture to another.

Foster (1976) categorised indigenous health practices of preliterate societies into two sub-systems. They are (i) personalistic and (ii) naturalistic systems. According to him in the personalistic system, the disease is explained as due to the 'active purposeful intervention of an agent, who may be human - a witch, or sorcerer, a non-human being - such as a spirit, an ancestor or evil spirit or supernatural being - a deity or other very powerful being. Lewis (1958) has noted that advantages of learning about indigenous beliefs and practices of a community lie in the insight it gives into a worldview of the people. The concept of disease causation (etiology) is one part of the societies total worldview which is also reflected in other spheres of life, such as agriculture, politics and interpersonal relations.

In contrast to the personalistic system, the naturalistic system explains illness in impersonal systematic terms. The disease is thought to stem, not from the machinations of an angry being but rather from such natural force or conditions as cold, heat, wind, dampness, and above all from an upset in the balance of the basic body elements. Health conforms to an equilibrium model causality concept in the naturalistic system, which explains or account for the upsets in the balance that trigger illness. The curative for a remedy in both the system is the identification of the spirits,

Gods causing illness, appeasing them by prayers, rituals, sacrifice, driving out an evil spirit from the body of the patient uttering spells, providing a device to protect against them, administration of herbal medicine and in some cases prescription of diet also. Thus, it seems that scientific system has developed from the naturalistic medical system.

The sick person literally is a victim, the object of aggression or punishment directed specifically against him, for reason that concern him alone (Foster and Anderson, 1978). Dubos (1969) opined that 'ancient medicine was the mother of science and played a large role in the integration of early cultures'. Thus, the scientific study of the medical system in a pre-literate society helps to find the rationale in the primitive concept of illness while controlling them to the modern medical system.

The medical system not directly derived from modern science is referred by different terms giving the same meaning as 'ethno medicine', 'folk-medicine', and 'popular health culture' (Erasmus, 1970). There is a great debate with regard to the use of word-traditional medicine while unfolding the indigenous method of handling of human illness. They opine herbal medicines used by indigenous people in general and the medicine men, in particular, are time tested, scientifically authenticated and have established to the assessment of medical field since time immemorial. They prefer the word contemporary medicine as a replacement for traditional medicine. It refers to the long-standing indigenous systems of healthcare found in the developing countries particularly among indigenous populations.

The paradigms of these indigenous medical systems view humanity as being intimately linked with the wider dimensions of nature. 'Indigenous medicine is a set of concepts of health and illness that reflect certain values, traditions, and beliefs based on the people's way of life, or culture' (Segesmundo, 1994) and its relevance to people's lives even as it only primarily responds to people's health problems.

In the bygone days the traditional medicine was considered as quackery and fringe, but now it is known as an alternative and complementary medicine. WHO has defined traditional medicine as a sum total of knowledge, skill, and practices based on the theories, beliefs, and experiences, indigenous to different cultures whether explicable or not, used on maintenance of health as well as in the prevention and diagnosis of diseases,, and improvement of treatment of physical and mental illness. Traditional medicine is an oral tradition purely empirical in nature that exists in all pre-literate and tribal communities. Notwithstanding technological advancement, traditional medicine still occupies a privileged place in the majority of the population in the Third World and life-threatening patients in the West. In addition, traditional medicine being cost effective and easily accessible, have been used since time immemorial and have passed the test of time without having side effects.

Studies on the indigenous medical system and healthcare practices of preliterate society, an important aspect of anthropology has a long history in different parts of the Globe. In most of the cases, it is very complex in nature and has components like beliefs, practices, rituals, and herbal medicine, spell, emulate, appeasing of deities, village medicine men and much more. In the domain of health issues of tribal populations, Indian Anthropologists have made some notable contribution, however, keeping in view the enormous diversity in tribal perception of health and illness and multitude of health problems that affect the tribes, and there is urgent need to explore the indigenous health practices and health seeking behaviour of the tribal communities. There is a lot to be understood and done with regard to tribal health in India.

The entire North East India provides shelter to numerous population groups of various ethnic affiliations having diverse social structures and cultural heritages. Due to the gradual adaptation to their respective environment, each population had developed their distinctive customs, values and belief system regarding the cause and cure of illness. In this treatise, we delve into the underlying causes of health disparities among indigenous population groups of North East India, a region with over two hundred forty different indigenous groups and a total population of 4,57,72,188 individuals. In this compilation, we could able to present only a snapshot through nineteen research contributions covering different regions and issues related to indigenous health practices.

The topics covered in the present treatise include indigenous notions of health, healer and healing practices prevailed in the region; ethnobotanical and ethnozoological knowledge; child-rearing practices; and reconciliation. It is hoped that the compilation would provide a better understanding towards the key determinants of the health and well-being of the indigenous people in the context of public health as there is a dearth of information assessing this relationship.

The traditional medicine needs protection and promotion on the part of the government otherwise, it may not compensate the healthcare services any longer. Attempt should be made to find a meaningful collaboration between indigenous and modern health systems.

References

Dubos R. 1968. *Man, Medicine and Environment*. Harmondsworth; Pelican.

Erasmus, CJ. 1970. 'Folk beliefs and relative of empirical knowledge'. *South Western Journal of Anthropology.* 8: 411-428.

Foster, George, and Barbara Gallatin Anderson. 1978. *Medical Anthropology*. New York; Wiley.

Foster, GM., 1976. 'Disease aetiologies in non-western medical systems'. *American Anthropologist*, 78, 4: 773-782.

Hasan, KA. 1967. *The Cultural Frontiers of Health in Village India: Case Study of a North Indian Village*. Mumbai; Manaktalas.

Lewis, A.1953. 'Health as a social concept'. In D. Mechank (Ed): *Readings in Medical Sociology*. pp. 113-127, New York; Free Press.

Segesmundo, MCL. 1994. 'Traditional health systems: Challenges in the Philippines'. pp. 110-114. In A. Islam and R. Wiltshire (Eds): *Traditional Health Systems and Public Policy*. Ottawa, Canada; International Development Research Centre

Siegerist, HE. 1951. *A History of Medicine*. Volume I, New York; Oxford University Press.

Dated: Dibrugarh 19 October 2017 **Sarthak Sengupta**

Acknowledgements

I personally owe a debt of profound gratitude to all those learned contributors for their academic cooperation in making my effort a reality. Without their kind academic help, this volume would not have seen the light of the day.

My wife Kaveeta, my wonderful sons Sushruta and Samrat deserve appreciation for their immeasurable poise, patience, and prop up. Thanks to my daughter-in-law Surovee who shielded me from that my granddaughter Shinjinee did not bother me too much during editing of the volume.

Professor Geeta Talukdar, FNA Sc, to whom this small treatise is being dedicated, was born on 28th July 1936. She obtained her MBBS (1957) and MD (1964) degrees from Delhi University and Ph.D. in Medicine (1967) from University of Kolkata. She had a luminous academic career, and was the recipient of Post Graduate Research Associate from CSIR and ICMR, New Delhi; trained at Karolinska Institute, Stockholm and Institute of Child Health, London; and served in Post Graduate Medical Education and Research, Kolkata; Vivekananda Institute of Medical Sciences, Kolkata. Professor Talukdar had written extensively – three well-knitted books on genetics, over 170 valuable research articles and successfully mentored 20 Ph.Ds who are now well established in their respective fields. I had the opportunity to work together with Geetadi as Co-Research Investigator in few Research projects sponsored to her by DBT and DST, Government of India and also accompanied with her in a number of field trips in some remote areas of North East India.

Professor Talukdar expired on 1st September 2008. To her, my debt of gratefulness is too enormous to be ever repaid. I humbly dedicate this work to her to express my deep sense of gratitude through unfathomable reverence.

Dated: Dibrugarh 19 October 2017 Sarthak Sengupta

List of Contributors

M. C. Arun, Department of Anthropology, Manipur University, Canchipur, Imphal, Manipur, 795 003.

K. N. Barua, Rain Forest Research Institute, Sotai, Jorhat, 785 001, Assam.

Somnath Bhattacharjee, Department of Anthropology, Assam University, Diphu, Karbi Anglong, 782 462, Assam.

Juri Borah, Department of Anthropology, Dibrugarh University, Dibrugarh, 786004, Assam,

S. K. Borthakur, Department of Botany, Gauhati University, Guwahati, Assam.

Mondira Borua, Department of Anthropology, Dibrugarh University, Dibrugarh, 786 004, Assam.

Dharmendra Changmai, Department of Anthropology Silapathar Science College, Silapathar, Dhemaji, Assam.

Tonjam Joshila Chanu, Department of Anthropology, Manipur University, Canchipur, Imphal, Manipur, 795 003.

Bhaskar Das, Department of Anthropology, D. H. S. K. College, Dibrugarh, 786 001, Assam.

Ratna Jyoti Das, Department of Pharmaceutical Sciences, Dibrugarh University, Dibrugarh, 786 004, Assam.

Anindita Deka, Department of Zoology, Arya Vidyapeeth College, Guwahati, 781016, Assam.

Purnima Devi, Department of Botany, Cotton College, Guwahati, 781001, Assam.

H.N. Dhungana, Rain Forest Research Institute, Sotai, Jorhat, 785 001, Assam.

Priya Dhungana, Department of Botany, Cotton College, Guwahati, 781 001, Assam.

Dali Dutta, Department of Anthropology, Dibrugarh University, Dibrugarh, 786 004, Assam.

S.K. Ghosh, Department of Pharmaceutical Sciences, Dibrugarh University, Dibrugarh, 786 004, Assam.

P.K. Hazarika, Rain Forest Research Institute, Sotai, Jorhat, 785 001, Assam.

Ranjumoni Hazarika, Department of Anthropology, Dibrugarh University, Dibrugarh, 786 004, Assam.

R.K. Kar, Department of Anthropology, Dibrugarh University, Dibrugarh, 786004, Assam.

Deepa Patir Changmai, Department of Anthropology, Silapathar Science College, Silapathar, Dhemaji, Assam.

Seema Pushkar, University Institute of Pharmacy, C.S.J.M. University, Kanpur, 208 024, Uttar Pradesh.

Melody Seb Rengma, Department of Anthropology, Dibrugarh University, Dibrugarh, 786 004, Assam.

Nikhil K. Sachan, University Institute of Pharmacy, C.S.J.M. University, Kanpur, 208 024, Uttar Pradesh.

Sarthak Sengupta, Department of Anthropology, Dibrugarh University, Dibrugarh, 786 004, Assam.

Samrat Sengupta, Department of Ecology and Environmental Science, Assam University, Silchar and Assistant Field Officer, Manas Landscape, Wildlife Trust of India, Sector-8, Noida, 201301, Uttar Pradesh.

Maitreyee Sharma, Department of Anthropology, Dibrugarh University, Dibrugarh, 786 004, Assam.

Haobijam Vokendra Singh, Department of Anthropology, Rajiv Gandhi University, Rono Hills, Doimukh, Itanagar, Papum Pare, 791112, Arunachal Pradesh.

Chandrajyoti Sonowal, Centre for Study of Social Inclusion and Inclusive Policies, Tata Institute of Social Sciences, Deonar, 400088, Mumbai.

Longkiri Timung, Department of Anthropology, Assam University, Diphu, Karbi Anglong, 782 462, Assam.

Sar-im Tisso, Department of Anthropology, Assam University, Diphu, Karbi Anglong, 782 462, Assam.

Kitoholi V. Zhimo, Department of Anthropology, University of Delhi, Delhi, 110 007, India.

Chapter - 1

Indigenous Knowledge System *Vis-à-Vis* Tribal Health Practices

—*R. K. Kar*

The entire field of Indigenous Knowledge system has attracted considerable attention in the recent past. An increasing number of global institutions (including UNESCO) are now concerned with defending, promoting and using Traditional Knowledge more widely. The relationship between Intellectual Property and Traditional Knowledge has been receiving increased attention in many policy fora and debates, ranging from food and agriculture, environment, health, human rights and cultural policy to trade and economic development. In recognition of its relevance and importance, National Institute of Science Communication (NISCOM), New Delhi, since around a decade has been publishing '*Indian Journal of Traditional Knowledge*' dealing exclusively with indigenous knowledge systems. Considering the resurgence of interest in ethnobotany as a source of new Pharmaceuticals, the first issue of the journal (2002) was devoted to deal exclusively with some studies in this field.

India, as a matter of fact, is considered as one of the greatest storehouses of traditional knowledge. She is blessed with a very rich and diverse heritage. Since time immemorial, the country has harboured and nurtured a variety of knowledge system.

Along with traditional knowledge system, India is also gifted with an immense wealth of rich bio-diversity that accounts for around eight per cent of the world's total biodiversity. According to an estimate, there are around 45,000 species of wild plants in India; and out of these around 7,500 species are in medical use in indigenous health practices (Vedavathy, 2002:25). The tribals who by and large, depend on forest wealth are the real custodians who safeguard the medicinal plants.

II

While dwelling specifically on Indigenous Knowledge and Health Practices, it may relevantly be noted that Disease and Ill-health has been one of the fundamental concerns of man since his emergence on the earth. Every known society has developed its own responses and methods for coping up with diseases and ailments, and eventually a body of its own medicinal system. "Medicine has been practiced one way or another since man became a cultural animal, there are even some evidence that a first aid technique derives from our primate ancestors ....baboons" (Clune, 1976:5, cited in Khan and Ali, 1992:11).

The disease-related beliefs and practices that are the products of indigenous cultural development; and are not explicitly derived from the conceptual framework of modern medicine constitute a distinct subdivision of *medical anthropology* which is known as *ethnomedicine*. Etymologically speaking, the term refers to the medicines that are traditionally associated with specific ethnic groups. Thus, it can also be conceived of as *Folk medicine*, *Traditional medicine* or *Indigenous medicine* etc. (Mibang and Choudhury, 2003:1).

It may contextually be noted here that beginning with their earliest field research around some 100 years ago, anthropologists, in a routine way have gathered data on the medical beliefs of the peoples, they studied, in the same way; and for the same purpose that they have gathered on all other aspects of culture to have as complete an ethnographic record as possible.

It was, however, the noted British Physician-cum-anthropologist W.H.R. Rivers (1924) who first developed the idea that indigenous medical system is social institutions to be studied in the same way as social institutions in general; and that indigenous medical practices are rational actions when viewed in the light of prevailing causation beliefs.

Incidentally, neither Rivers nor Clements (1932) nor any of their contemporaries, engaged in collecting data on primitive medical systems had any idea that they were doing medical anthropological research, and they seemed to have been unconcerned with the possible significance of their findings to the health of the people, they studied. Consequently, we cannot say that medical anthropology has developed out of early research on primitive medicine. Rather, it is the another way round. Anthropologists, working in the health fields today have, in fact, recaptured and given a formal name ethnomedicine to the study of traditional non-western medicine, and made it a part of their specialty.

As medical anthropology has developed, especially in the broad areas of international public health and trans-cultural Psychiatry, the theoretical importance of knowledge about non-western medical systems has become apparent. This recognition has sparked renewed interest in ethnomedicinal research, elevating it to a very important exercise in medical anthropology.

III

The subject of ethnomedicine, in fact, focuses on the nature of illness as it is conceived by the natives; their own methods; criteria of classification of diseases; the causes and cures; types of therapists and healers who seek to alleviate illness, and their skills and social roles; preventive measures; the relation between medicine and religion; cultural aspects of medicine and also ethno-psychiatry (Hughes, 1968 and Foster, 1978). The primary concern of ethnomedicine is thus with the description of notions, people have about health and illness and about the behaviour they undertake in search of cures.

Rubel (1977:120) explains the concept of illness as syndromes from which members of a particular group claim to suffer and for which their culture provides etiology, diagnosis, preventive measures and regimes of healing. Studies of the relationship between health and harmony in the beliefs of the Navaho (Adair *et al.,* 1957); and of the moral implications attributed to the illness of several cultures (Fabrega, 1972), for example, provide ample demonstrations of the socio-cultural bearing on the notions of health and illness.

Data collected through the ethnomedicinal approach contribute, not only to the understanding of medical systems in their cultural contents but also lend insight into the understanding of the interface between the indigenous and western medical systems that affect socio-cultural change. The anthropologically oriented medical knowledge would be of immense use as an input to benefit disease control programmes and international health planning. Many of the disease control programmes have been introduced into areas where indigenous systems are yet strong; there have been great resistances (Khan and Ali, 1992:14).

An in-depth study of folk medicine also helps to find out the forces of integration and resistance with regard to the implementation of certain modern medical programmes. Once we come to understand the cultural forces that hinder the successful implementation of the programmes, it will not be difficult to work out and modify the framework of the programmes according to the suitability of the culture or community for which they are meant.

Also by going into an in-depth understanding of indigenous materia medica and pharmacopeia of various traditional cultures, it is possible in ethnomedicinal studies to discover the medicinal value of plants and animals which are so far unknown or least known to the modern world.

The pharmacopeia of folk medicines is copious and includes such proven drugs as quinine, opium, Drosera, thuja, and curare etc. Sometimes, the same species of plant is used for a host of purposes. Thus, for example, almost all the parts of the *Mahua* (*Madhuca longifolia*) plant are used by the tribals of Madhya Pradesh in various ailments and diseases; the root paste is given to treat stomach ulcer; it is applied on scorpion sting; the bark decoction is gargled in case of gum swelling; the decoction with that of *Ficus recemosa* is used for leucorrhoea; the bark is astringent and tonic; its decoction is given in diabetes and rheumatic diseases; the flowers are given in bronchitis and cough; the flower paste is applied to take out the pierced thorn; the fruit paste is applied in a toothache; the seed oil is massaged over the chest in the treatment of pneumonia; and the seed cake is used in snake bite; few drops of its decoction are put in the nostrils which result into vomiting and relief (Sikarwar, 2002:90).

When we focus our discourse, particularly in the context of tribal communities, it may be noted that the practice of ethnomedicine in the form of magical cures has usually an explicit social implication reflecting socially cohesive results. Typically, the curative session involves not only the patient and the healer but also the patient's family, clan members, and other neighbours. The curative rituals serve, in various ways, as an occasion for re-integration of the group around common social values. "Especially in societies lacking strong centralised socio-political institution, the occurrence and imminence of disease with the belief that it represents punishment for aberrant, dissocial impulse or action can be functionally important in maintaining group cohesion and restraining disruptive tendencies" (Sills, 1972:91).

IV

Because of a culturally and geographically diverse landscape, the north-east region of India exhibits a rich array of ethnomedicinal practices. But these have not been documented from several areas. Some piece-meal studies, however, have been reported in a number of professional journals and edited books (e.g. Choudhury, 1986, 1990; Mibang and Choudhury, 2003; Kalla and Joshi, 2004).

The region provides shelter to numerous peoples of various ethnic affiliations having different social structures, cultural heritages and cultural linkages across the international borders. There is a rich assembly of tribal cultures and communities in this rugged expanse of the eastern Himalayas. There are more than 140 major tribal groups in North East India, having quite a good number of sub-tribes. In other words, around one-third of the total numbers of listed tribes for the whole of India is to be found in this region. The percentage of the tribal population in different states ranges from 11 (Assam) to 94 (Mizoram). The average percentage of the tribal population in the region is 22 (Kar, 2001).

Though the traditional outlook, customs, rituals, beliefs, habits, and concepts of etiology, as well as diagnosis and treatment of diseases, are changing fast under the impact of an ongoing modernisation process, a number of studies, carried out among various tribal groups of North East India (e.g, among the Boro Kacharis - Guha, 1986 a and 1986b; Idu Mishmis - Dutta Choudhury and Ghosh, 1984; Kaman Mishmis - Barua, 1984; Koch Rajbanshis – Guha, 1990; Pnars - Bhatt, 1986; Singphos - Dutta Choudhury, 1985; and the Noctes – Kar, 1993; Kar and Gogoi, 1993, 1994) reveal that in most of the tribal and rural societies traditional health behaviours not only dominate over the modern ones but also very often hinder the acceptance of the latter. The people, by and large, are dependent on nature. The healing system is thus intimately connected with the cosmos, emic perceptions of different natural phenomena and belief in spirits.

V

While dwelling some more on the indigenous health practices and the tribals as a whole, it may be highlighted that the tribal medicines are the product of a gainful utilisation of the tribal medicinal heritage. Since time immemorial, they have been using herbs, minerals and other substances in treating their sick patients. They also have knowledge of physiotherapy, childbirth, and gynecology. The entire medicinal heritage of the tribals can thus probably be considered as an alternative system of therapy. Anthropologists and Botanists have amassed a vast amount of data on ethnomedicines. In any case, the tribal claims of their medicines need to be verified scientifically.

Incidentally, the tribal systems of medicine have been characterised as magico-religious for the simple reason that the elements of magic and religion greatly influenced the proceedings of these systems. The disease causation theory in the systems takes its main inspiration from the culturally postulated supernatural forces and agents which are believed to be intricately linked to the human world. A disease of a person may be conceptualised as merely a projection of the wrath of supernatural entities; and therefore, the intervention of medicines may not be considered necessary and desirable by the people.

The shaman, sorcerer, priest, *Ojha,* and *Bej* etc., are the human agents having the capacity to intervene and mediate in the events of supernatural encounters. In this context, Joshi (2004:403-407) raises a pertinent issue, "what should be done if the tribals subscribe to the magico-religious world view? Should we act as social reformers and teach them that their beliefs and practices are all hocus-pocus, and they should stop believing in them? In order to do this, we will first have to make sure that we provide them with an effective and guaranteed alternative." He further continues, "The problem [however] does not end here, we will also have to know the clinical and social importance of the tribal magico-religious practices....... The significance of magico-religious practices in the reduction of anxiety, neurosis, phobias, stress and other psychopathological conditions have to be clinically evaluated. Beyond all these, the contribution of magico-religious ritual which often involves a large group and has a much therapeutic effect through public singing, trance and catharsis should also be ascertained."

As a matter of fact, the tribal system of medicine, as noted earlier, invariably involves the community in the therapy; and this is a great strength of the system. Incidentally, our hospitals and health centre lack social milieu; and the entire approach is contractual, formal and individualistic.

The social support network in health seeking process provides an implicit reassurance to the patient and his immediate dependents. The therapy, therefore, becomes a group concern. The experience of sickness thereby becomes a shared experience. In such a scenario, the rehabilitation of the patient is never a problem; and the stigma of a disease is a non-entity. The importance of social milieu becomes extremely relevant in the event of severe mental illness and disability. In the matter of social support, we, the urbanites have much to learn from the tribal systems.

VI

According to a study carried out by the United Nations Development Programme, "Eighty per cent of the world's population depends on indigenous knowledge to meet their medical needs......" (Down to Earth, 1996, p. 3. cited in Mibang and Chaudhuri, 2003:5). In the context of health, disease, and medical treatment, Agarwal (1996:53) laments, "It is a matter of great concern that India lacks a health policy worth the name.

Nearly, a billion people have no assured access to healthcare and the benefits of modern science……. Besides traditional diseases, new diseases are cropping up due to changing lifestyles and deteriorating environmental conditions."

He continues, "…….the challenge before us today is: how do we develop low-cost medicine to deal with our health problem? The two major ways to reduce costs are preventive health programmes and traditional curative care….." Traditional (ethnic) medicine, as a matter of fact, can play a very important role in providing low-cost services.

The modern Medicare services are not only very expensive but also have their alarming adverse side effects. In search of a real alternative, we need to remember that the mother of all indigenous medicines is the tribal medicine, practiced by the communities living in close harmony with the ecosystem. There is thus an urgent need for documentation of not only the herbal medicines but also the tribal health practices in totality. There is also an urgent need to translate all the available traditional knowledge as per international standards and safeguard the patenting rights of the stakeholders. It should, however, be remembered that if the documentation is to be of value in modern drug discovery programme, it is to be done in relatively more details with respect to the information like symptoms, methods of indigenous preparation, dosages, sources of information, modes of administration and the final outcome of the treatment.

References

Adair, John; Kurt Denschle and Mc Dermott. 1957. 'Some problems of the physicians on the Navaho reservation'. *Human Organisation*. 16: 19-23.

Agarwal, A. 1996. 'To be healthy, wealthy and wise'. *Down to Earth*, June 15.

Barua, S. 1984. 'A study on indigenous health practices among the Kaman Mishmis of Lohit district of Arunachal Pradesh'. *Human Science*, 33: 332-344.

Bhatt, KH. 1986. 'Concept of health and disease among the Pnars of Meghalaya', in B. Chaudhuri (Ed): *Tribal Health: Socioeconomic Dimensions*. pp. 259-274, New Delhi; Inter-India Publications.

Chaudhury, B. 1986. *Tribal Health: Socioeconomic Dimensions*. New Delhi; Inter-India Publications.

Chaudhury, B.1990. *Cultural and Environmental Dimensions of Health*. New Delhi; Inter-India Publications.

Clements, FE. 1932. 'Primitive concepts of disease'. *American Archaeology and Ethnology*, 32:185-252.

Dutta Choudhury, SS. 1985. 'Herbal medicine and its implication in family planning: A study based upon the Singpho of Arunachal Pradesh'. *Human Science*, 34: 75-77.

Dutta Choudhury, SS, and GC. Ghosh, 1994. 'Indigenous health practices among the Idu Mishmis of Arunachal Pradesh'. *Human Science*, 33: 24-34.

Fabrega, Horacio Jr.,1972. 'Medical Anthropology', In BJ. Siegel (Ed): *Biennial Review of Anthropology*. Stanford, California; Stanford University Press.

Foster, George, and Barbara Gallatin Anderson. 1978. *Medical Anthropology*. New York; Wiley.

Guha, A., 1986a. 'Folk Medicine of the Boro Kacharis- A Plains tribe of Assam', in B. Chaudhuri (Ed): *Tribal Health: Sociocultural Dimensions*. pp. 191-200. New Delhi; Inter-India Publications.

Guha, A., 1986b. 'Herbs in the disease treatment by Bodo Kachari- A Plains tribe of Assam'. *Journal Indian Anthropological Society*, 21:219-230.

Guha, A., 1990. 'Health care among two rural populations of Assam: A comparative study', In B. Chaudhuri (Ed): *Cultural and Environmental Dimensions of Health*. pp. 207-248. New Delhi; Inter-India Publications.

Hughes, Charles C., 1968. 'Ethnomedicine'. In *International Encyclopedia of Social Sciences*, New York; Free Press, Macmillan.

Joshi, PC, 2004. 'Issues in tribal health and medicines', In AK. Kalla and PC. Joshi (Ed): *Tribal Health and Medicines*. pp. 403-407, New Delhi; Concept Publishing Company.

Kalla, AK, and PC. Joshi, 2004. *Tribal Health and Medicine*. New Delhi; Concept Publishing Company.

Kar, RK, 1993. 'Reproductive health behavior of the Nocte women in Arunachal Pradesh'. *Social Change*, 23, 4: 40-52.

Kar, RK, 2001. 'Anthropological appraisal of a migrant population in Assam, North East India'. *Presidential Address, Anthropology and Archaeology Section,* 88th Session of Indian Science Congress. New Delhi, 3-7 January 2001.

Kar, RK and Juri Gogoi, 1993. 'Health status of the Noctes of Arunachal Pradesh'. *Social Change*, 23: 164-171.

Kar, RK and Juri Gogoi, 1994. 'Morbidity in an Arunachal Pradesh tribe: Some field notes from a Nocte Village'. *Resarun*, 18:133-142.

Khan, CG, and Md. Arif Ali, 1992. 'Relevance of ethnomedicine'. *Man and Life,* 18:11-20.

Mibang, Tamo, and SK. Chaudhuri, 2003. *Ethno Medicines of the Tribes of Arunachal Pradesh.* Delhi; Himalayan Publisher.

Rivers, WHR, 1924. *Medicine, Magic, and Religion*. New York; Har Court Brace.

Rubel, J Arthur, 1977. 'The Epidemiology of folk illness: Susto in Hispanic America', In David Landy (Ed): *Culture, Disease, and Healing*. New York; McMillan Publishing Corporation Inc.

Sills, DS, 1972. *International Encyclopedia of Social Sciences*. New York; Free Press.

Vedavathy, S. 2002. 'Tribal medicine: The real alternative'. *Indian Journal of Traditional Knowledge*, 1, 1:25-31.

Chapter - 2

Revisiting the Domain of Ethnomedicine: Some Issues and Methods

—C. J. Sonowal

As it appears the term 'ethnomedicine' is composed of two words– 'ethno' and 'medicine'. The word ethnos is defined as 'nation'. The related term 'ethnic' refers currently to people thought to have common ancestry who share a distinctive culture. Within the social sciences, however, the usage has become more generalised to all human groups that explicitly regard themselves and are regarded by others as culturally distinctive. Among the first to bring the term 'ethnic group' into social studies was the German sociologist Max Weber, who defined it (1922) as:

> *Those human groups that entertain a subjective belief in their common descent because of similarities of physical type or of customs or both, or because of memories of colonisation and migration; this belief must be important for group formation; furthermore, it does not matter whether an objective blood relationship exists.*

The word 'medicine' that follows the word 'ethnic' stands for a different meaning from its usual and very objective connotation. For example, in American Anthropological literature the 'medicine' in 'ethnomedicine' usually refers to knowledge and ideas about health and healthcare. It may mean medication or treatment practices in European and biological literature. In fact, the term medicine has several related definitions dealing with health and well-being—physical, physiological and psychological. Therefore, when one talks of medicine of any particular culture, they simply refer to the ethnomedicine of that culture.

Components in Ethnomedicine

Generally speaking, ethnomedicine is the area of anthropology that studies different society's notions of health and illness, their perception, and actions related to health and well-being. Equipped with the shield of 'ethnic' the branch of ethnomedicine deals with the issues of health and well-being in an 'emic' perspective – that is the perspective of the members of the particular culture. But the quite interesting aspect of such issue is that these 'emic' components mostly become visible or understandable through 'etic' discourse only. This is because most of such behaviours appear '*normal*' or '*taken for granted*' which leaves behind little space for scientific investigation and analysis leading to explanation.

Ethnomedicine seeks to understand the base of a culture's common sense or medical logic that people use to explain and treat their illness. This, it does, by examining the health-related theories and knowledge that people inherit and learn by living in a culture. Next, ethnomedicine is not simply the static and isolated study of single cultures. Comparing and translating the underlying aspects of every such ethnomedicinal study can lead to the applicability of such knowledge in improved and effective healthcare delivery in diverse world.

Importance of Combining Ethnomedicine and Biosciences

Translating the emic behaviour (ethnomedicine) into etic ways is important so as to convert belief and perception into action towards better health. This process is important in the contemporary world of health and well-being in that diseases are penetrating across different cultural domains creating varied forms of illness and emerging challenges to the local and global communities. In this situation, the effectiveness, applicability, and acceptability of a particular healthcare system (ethnomedicine) remain crucial one. *Medical pluralism* has proved to be a better option, especially in traditional societies at least among those who are exposed to the non-traditional domain to a certain extent.

Browner *et al.* (1988) propose that emic perspective of ethnomedicine may be combined with the etic perspective of bioscience in the following ways:

(i) Identify the health problems and how it is conceivably healed according to locals.

(ii) Objectively assess the remedy's ability to produce the emically desired effect.

(iii) Identify the areas of convergence and divergence between the emic and etic assessments.

Arthur Kleinman (1980) forwards the 'explanatory model' (EM) by saying that people try to integrate more than one aspects related to the illness they encounter centreing around the popular illness ideologies– the idiosyncratic thoughts and circumstances, current in their culture. These may include the potential cause of illness, its effect and the way to make it better. Kleinman asserts that culture influences the construction of EM through theories and explanatory themes and images. These are manifested in the terms and languages used while describing different aspects of illness–infecting, resisting, possessing, fighting etc.

Cultural ideas about the nature of the body and illness, the cultural philosophies about morality, responsibility, autonomy, powerful forces etc converge to form an ethnomedical system. This he terms as 'internal logic' which may be viewed differently by the different cultural entity.

The understanding of ethnomedicine is also closely related to certain issues like body image, ethnic-physiology etc. People in society have different concepts about the body which may be termed as 'body image'. It determines what, when, where and how a body should behave, accept or respond to certain conditions and how do they respond to illness condition. Likewise, there are also perceived physiological norms and beliefs that interpret various physiological aspects of the human body (for example menstruation) having a significant effect on health and treatment seeking behaviour.

Anthropology of Health: Positivist and Interpretive Dichotomy

Early medical anthropologists defined health as 'a broad construct, consisting of physical, physiological and social well-being including role functionality. Later on, by the year 1970, distinctions between 'disease' and 'illness' was proposed. Accordingly, it has been conceived that 'disease' is a bio-medically measurable lesion or anatomical or physiological irregularities and 'illness' is the culturally structured, personal experience of being unwell, which entails the experience of suffering. This dichotomy also put the issue in the positivist vs. interpretive dichotomy that goes as follows:

Etic - Disease - Body: Essentially objective and universally similar so positivist.

Emic – Illness - Mind: Essentially specific to a certain culture and varied and interpretive in nature.

It has also been theorised that both disease and illness can be located in person. But, there is a distinction. Though disease may persist in a particular body, illness manifest only when a condition, out of disease, makes the body unable to fulfill social roles and relations of varied nature.

The Bio-cultural Nature of Ethnomedicine

Any study on ethnomedicine of a particular culture must deal with socio-physical and socio-psychological and cultural aspects. This is because the health and treatment seeking behaviour of the members of that culture are intertwined with their long-standing perception about cause-effect relations influenced by cultural thoughts. Therefore, enumerating or recording of healthcare and treatment alone is not sufficient to depict the complete ethnomedical domain in a community. Behind every behaviour and practice, the meaning the people put on it is of utmost importance for a single as well as the cross-cultural study of ethnomedicine.

Biomedical domain very often assigns folk knowledge as only a belief system, devoid of objective or empirical reality. Minus the medical property of Ethnomedicine, it says, all are just psycho-social concepts nothing to do with the diseases people encounter with. Here comes the very crucial relationship between human body and mind–mind, here, a moulded entity by culture and society where the body lives.

While the discourse on body and mind is made it is quite essential to differentiate between *healing and cure*. These two terms are essential to understanding the components of the ethnomedicine of any given society. It is quite often asserted that 'cure' denotes physical removal of any health condition. Thus, once cured the condition should no longer be there in the body. Healing, on the other hand, is mostly a psychological state of mind possessed by a diseased body. Healing is a broader perception in that it influences both body and the mind. A diseased body may be cured physically, but unless the healing process is not complete illness may not go completely. Contrarily, a person may not be cured of the physical ailment. But healing can positively influence the mind of the person in such a way that he may no longer be an ill person. He may accept the physical condition as a normal state of happening in life course and adapt to that state of life. He or the society is likely to create a situation in and around him conducive to his physicality so that he performs his culturally assigned or perceived roles and relations. This explains why a very ill person or a dying person in traditional societies invites fellow people, performs rituals, shares its views and gets ready to die with grace. These are the healing process in traditional societies which make the affected person feel that his physical condition is no longer an illness. Rather it is the condition manifested as a result of certain acts or eventualities which he cannot, probably, get rid of and he is destined to get it. This gives him willpower and logical justification to deal with the situation and he is no longer afraid of the ultimate result of the condition.

In the same way, many curable diseases affect people in an incurable or chronic way due to the absence of such healing process. This healing process may be anything ranging from social support, a rational explanation of cause-effect relations, and a ritual, folk way of listening to myths and legends and so on. The folkways of ethnomedicine domain are full of such healing process in the form of rites and rituals, magico-religious practices and prescribed personal ways of care and behaviour etc. There are numerous such examples in tribal societies. Besides utilisation of herbal components, folk medicines are attached with lots of description prescription modalities towards use, observances, and follow-ups. For instance, among the traditional Sonowal Kacharis, when a person becomes ill, the first and the foremost initiative will be to tie a packet (*tupula*) consisting of betel nut and betel leaf in the name of the household deity. Subsequently, according to the symptom of the illness, the related deities are remembered and the packets of betel nuts are tied and fix it to the ceiling of the house. If it is felt that any rituals have to be performed then and there, it is done. Otherwise, the people have a fixed timeline throughout the year to perform related rituals. After using a home remedy or traditional medicine (if available) if the problem persists, the head of the family takes permission from the household deity to take the ill person out for further treatment with alien medicine. These activities offer the people a sense of security from supernatural beings and believe that the malevolent influence leaves the body and the benevolent deities clear the body for physical treatment.

The significance of all these behaviour lies in the fact that the ill person and the family are now free from all sort of fear that they have been influenced by any benevolent or malevolent power. It remains now only a matter of physical issue which may or may not be cured. But the person is mentally prepared to face it without a dual state of mind. So he is already healed. People believe that medicine does not work in a possessed body because the possessing power only consumes or destroy the effect of the medicine applied to a possessed body. The harmony of body and mind is the pre-requisite in all sort of treatment system, including biomedical domain.

It is evident that such rationalisation does not require for the part of the people who follow such behaviour simply because culture and tradition give a strong and undeniable platform to act accordingly, ultimately serving the purpose for them. Nothing is meaningless in a given culture if behaviours in question are adopted by most of its members. Rather, quite a few of such behaviours have direct relation even with biomedical empiricism. For example, the cleanliness observed by the most of the traditional tribal societies during the appearance of chicken pox in any member of the family, or sometimes anybody in the village and the rules of maintaining utmost calm and silence etc in the village is also explainable in biomedical system, for the disease attracts risk of infection in dirty environment and mental disturbance increases irritation in patients increasing severity of the disease.

Importance of Investigation on Health and Treatment Seeking Behaviour

These delineations indicate that a meaningful and effective ethnomedicinal study should reflect all such aspects so as to make it applicable cross-culturally. Studying of the presence of traditional medicine practices is not enough to make such study compatible in the contemporary situation. It is quite important how the people within the system respond to internal and external healthcare and treatment facilities and systems. Without such an understanding the entire knowledge level becomes static and stereotypic and is unable to answer several queries related to people's healthcare and treatment seeking behaviour in a pluralistic medical system. Therefore, to relate these aspects some methodological inquiries are needed, a part of which can be delineated here for instance.

Investigating Treatment Seeking Behaviour

The recent anthropological thinking about health seeking behaviour contrasts with its earlier '*cultural belief system*'. Now in addition to ideational or belief system, an *ecological framework* has been considered which emphasises a set of causal elements like environmental features, material/economic constraints, and political considerations. In such framework actors (the people) are not merely passive followers of cultural wisdom, rather they can choose and decide the course of behaviours selecting from a range of alternatives. The cultural knowledge in relation to illness now is seen as the rules or criteria for deciding among different possible actions.

Thus, the ecological perspective of health promotion approach is very much in practice in the present scenario. There are two basic premises on the basis of which intervention points can be identified.

(i) Behaviour affects and gets affected by multiple levels of influence.

(ii) Individual behaviour shapes and is shaped by social environment, which can be termed as the reciprocal of causation.

Two models have been discussed here among the host of models used by social scientists and public health professional in looking health seeking behaviour of people and community.

The Health Belief Model (HBM)

This is possibly the most known model in public health, and also the oldest one from social psychology, developed in the 1950s. Sheeran and Abraham (1995) present HBM on the basis of following factors and principles:

Beliefs about the impact of illness and its consequences (threat perception) which depend on:

- Perceived susceptibility, or the beliefs about how vulnerable a person considers him or herself in relation to a certain illness or health problem.
- Perceived severity of illness or health problems and its consequences;
  - (a) Health motivation or readiness to be concerned about health matters.
  - (b) Beliefs about the consequences of health practices and about the possibilities and the effort to put them into practice. The behavioural evaluation depends on:
    - Perceived benefits of preventive or therapeutic health practices;
    - Perceived barriers, both material and psychological, with regard to a certain health practice.
  - (c) Cues to action, which includes different, internal and external factors, which influence action. For example, nature and intensity (organic and symbolic) of illness symptoms, mass media campaigns, advice from relevant other (family, friends, health staff, etc.).
  - (d) Beliefs and health motivation are conditioned by socio-demographic variables (class, age, gender, religion, etc.) and by the psychological characteristics of the interviewed person (personality, peer group pressure etc).

The Health Belief Model (HBM)

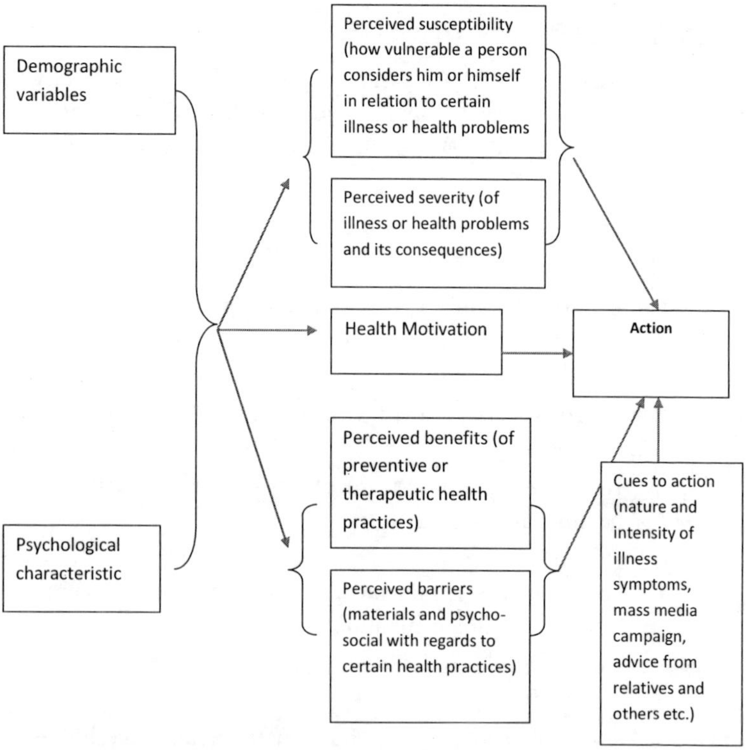

The Healthcare Utilisation Model

The socio-behavioural or Andersen model (Andersen and Newman, 1973) groups in a logic sequence three clusters or categories of factors (*predisposing*, *enabling* and *need* factors) which can influence health behaviour. The model was specifically developed to investigate the use of biomedical health services.

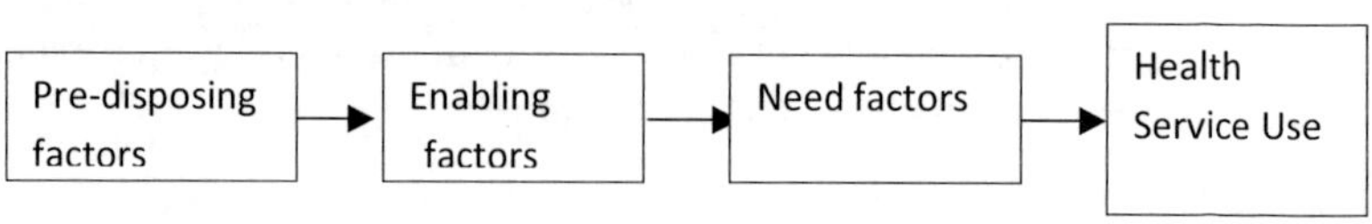

A further variant of Andersen's model was elaborated by Kroeger (1983). Based on an extensive and well-elaborated literature revision, he proposed the following framework:

Interrelated explanatory variables, all of which are affected by perceived morbidity.

(i) An individual's traits or predisposing factors: age, sex, marital status, status in the household, household size, ethnic group, the degree of cultural adaptation, formal education, occupation, assets (land, livestock, cash, income), social network interactions.

(ii) Characteristics of the disorder and their perception: chronic or acute, severe or trivial, etiological model, expected benefits or treatment (modern versus traditional), psychosomatic versus somatic disorders.

(iii) Characteristics of the service (health service system factors and enabling factors): accessibility, appeal (opinions and attitudes towards traditional and modern healers), acceptability, quality, communication, costs.

The interaction of these factors guides the selection of healthcare resources (dependent variables).

The Healthcare Utilization Model expanded by Kroeger, 1983

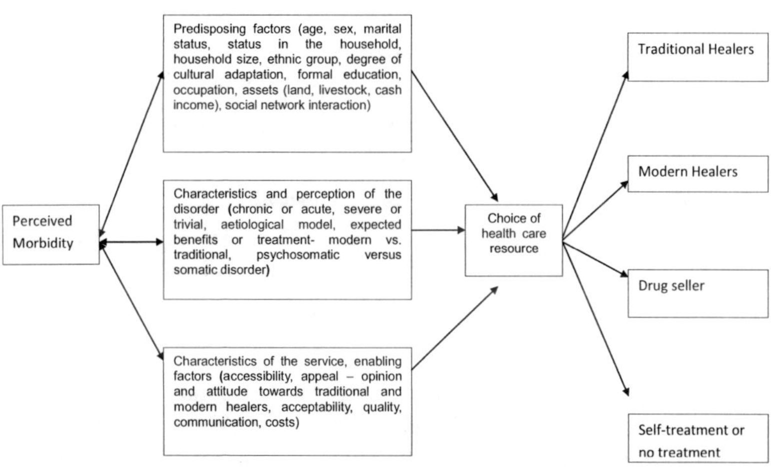

Research Questions

Some of the relevant research questions regarding an inquiry into the domain of Ethnomedicine in present day context may be listed as follows:

(i) What are the perception of health and illness in the traditional setting of the tribe?

(ii) What are the existing cultural norms, values, and belief in relation to treatment seeking behaviour among the selected people?

(iii) What is the nature and extent of their knowledge about the biomedical terminology of illness and diseases?

(iv) What are nature and extent of their knowledge and belief on curing and healing?

(v) What are the available healthcare facilities (traditional and modern system) among the selected people?

(vi) What are their knowledge and awareness on traditional and modern healthcare?

(vii) What are the healthcare programmes sponsored by government and NGOs?

(viii) In what way the availability and non-availability of resources like money, accessibility etc. have influenced their treatment seeking behaviour?

(ix) What is the nature and extent of interaction among factors like traditional beliefs and practices, physical environment and accessibility, affordability, awareness and availability/non-availability of modern healthcare facilities etc?

(x) What are the determinants that link perception and action in health and treatment seeking?

Focused Ethnographic Study (FES) Method

In ethnomedicinal studies, it is advisable to synthesise an in-depth survey-cum-observation of demographic and socio-cultural and political-economic environment of the studied population confined to the selected areas and utilisation of Focused Ethnographic Study (FES) method.

The FES method evolved as a result of a collaborative development work of applied anthropologists and public health specialists through which study guidelines were designed combining anthropological theory and techniques with rapid, focused data collection aimed at yielding clear and comprehensive recommendations apt for implementation. Important examples of such study guidelines are the Focused Ethnographic Studies (FES) developed for Acute Respiratory Infection (ARI) programme by Cove and Pelto (1994) and the Rapid Assessment Manual for Malaria (Akua Agyepond *et al.,* 1995).

With particular emphasis on qualitative methods, FES uses a variety of techniques. Key informant interview and case study are two basic techniques of data collection to be used in the study. Some of the basic aspects FES uses are as follows:

(i) An inquiry into the prevalence of various biomedically defined and locally known illness and their terms along with concerned signs and symptoms of a particular illness defined locally and listing them with the help of key informants etc.

(ii) Recording of locally perceived causes, progression, the degree of severity assigned to these symptoms.

(iii) Induction of a hypothetical scenario (vignettes) of illness to informants to enquire about normative behaviour against those illnesses. For example, the informant may be asked what will be the action if the illness is perceived as serious and economic resources are available or unavailable. Answers are quantified in percentages. Derived from the responses a series of rules are elaborated. For instance, one may drive into the rule that '*if a family has money and a severe illness occurs, they would consult a doctor*'.

(iv) The narrative about recent illness episodes and care seeking to show actual behaviour may be recorded. The recording of actual cases or 'episodes' of illness which in turn helps compare respondent's cultural or normative statement like beliefs about symptoms and illness with the behaviour they are engaging in, like treatment seeking.

(v) A continuous evaluation of findings and inputs of new orientations depending on results should follow.

(vi) An inquiry into the aspects like etiology (causes of diseases), the onset of symptoms, physiopathology (the mechanism by which diseases cause), the course of sickness (severity etc) and treatment.

(vii) The 'Healthcare system features' including obstacles like poor performance of health services, lack of drugs, economic factors, and decision-making power for healthcare within households can be inquired.

(viii) It is advisable to focus on a particular and defined area of illness at a time (not on all knowledge of illness in general) to explore the elements of knowledge/beliefs people bring to bear in specific instances or episode. It is expected that the key informant interview and analysis of cases will lead to a description of the explanation for a particular class or category of illness.

(ix) Ranking and ordering of signs, symptoms, and illness may be done with the help of key informants and respondents groups based on different perspectives like severity, reasons etc.

(x) After listing the emic terms of illness and also biomedical ones, the informant may be presented with the selected illness (to be examined), one at a time, and may be asked to select all the signs/symptoms that he/she considers to be associated with that illness. This assignment of signs/symptoms to individual 'illness' will form the early explanatory model for that illness.

(xi) A manageable number of illness may be considered for the FES on the basis of the classification made ranging from most severe to least severe (as perceived) curable either bio-medically or with the help of traditional practices or both.

Use of Theoretical Sampling

The theoretical base of treatment seeking behaviour among the tribal people has not been well built so far. Thus, it is apparent that we need some grounded theories to be built based on diverse ethnographic studies on ethnomedicine. For such a purpose theoretical sampling process is one of the best-known ways.

Theoretical sampling is a process of data collection by *evolving theory* and not directed by any *pre-determined* theory. It is based on certain concept indicator models of analysis—employing the method of constant comparison of cases or events. Defining theoretical sampling it can be said that it is a sampling procedure where selection or sampling of additional incidents, events, activities etc is directed by the evolving theoretical construct. It is a process 'where analyst jointly collects, codes, and analysis his data and decides what data to collect next and where to find them in order to develop his theory as it emerges' (Glaser, 1978).

The basic premises of grounded theory are as follows:

(i) Empirical indicators from the data (action and events–observed, recorded or described) are compared looking at similarities and dissimilarities.

(ii) The underlying uniformities of indicators are identified and a 'coded category' or concepts are formed.

(iii) Such concepts are compared with more empirical indicators and with other concepts so built thereby sharpening the definition of the concept and to define its properties.

(iv) Theories are formed from proposing probable relationship among concepts and sets of concepts.

(v) Tentative theories or theoretical propositions are further explained through additional instances of data.

Through theoretical sampling testing and comparison of additional information, cases etc go on continuously until additional analysis no longer contributes to anything new about a concept. In this way, the resulting

The Teoretical Sampling Guide (Adapted from Claire B. Draucker *et.al.,* 2007)

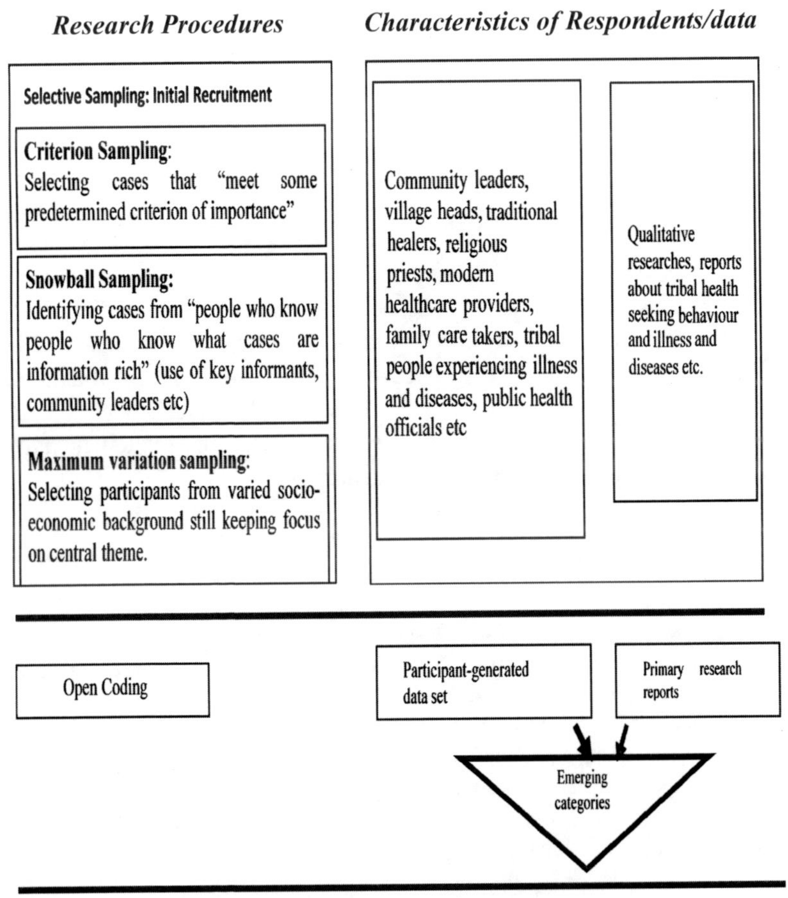

theory is considered conceptually dense and grounded in the data. Sampling in Grounded Theory is a sequential process. It has, to begin with, '*selective sampling*' and move into '*theoretical sampling*' when concepts begin to emerge. The definite coding process is intimately related to particular sampling procedure and particular types of activities related to data collection in theoretical sampling procedure.

References

Akua Agyepong, Irene.; B. Aryee; H.Dzikunu and L. Manderson. 1995. *The Malaria Manual: Guidelines for the Rapid Assessment of Social, Economic and Cultural Aspects of Malaria*. Geneva: World Health Organisation.

Anderson, R and JF Newman. 1973 ' Societal and individual determinants of medical care utilisation in the United States'. *The Milbank Memorial Fund Quarterly, Health and Society*. 51,1 : 95-124.

Browner, CH.; BRO de Montellano and AJ Rubel. 1988. 'A methodology for cross-cultural ethnomedical research'. *Current Anthropology*. 29, 5:681-702.

Cove, A and GH Pelto. 1994. 'Focused ethnographic studies in WHO programme for the control of acute respiratory infections'. *Medical Anthropology*. 15: 409-424.

Glasser, JW. 1978 'The effect of predation on prey resource utilisation'. *Ecology*. 59, 4: 724–732.

Kleinman, A. 1980. *Patients and Healers in the Context of Culture*. Barkley: University of California Press.

Kroeger, A. 1983. 'Anthropological and socio-medical health research in developing countries'. *Social Science and Medicine*. 17, 3: 147-161.

Weber, Max. 1922. 'Ethnic groups'. In Werner Sollars (Ed): *Theories of Ethnicity: A Classical Reader*. p. 52, New York: New York University Press.

Chapter - 3

Cross-cultural Comparison of Ethnozoological Treatments among the Tribes of North East India

—Haobijam Vokendro Singh

Introduction

Human beings in course of their evolution to different stages at different places of the world encountered different health and health-related problems- disease, sickness, and infirmities. From time immemorial, they have been attempting to solve such unavoidable health problems by employing different means and methods. Medical anthropology is such a sub-specialised field of inquiry of anthropology for understanding the holistic approach of health and health-related matters by synthesising both biological and cultural components of health and disease of the people in the past and at present of different communities of different parts of the world. The different ways and means of controlling and curing of ailments by using plants, animals and magico-religious therapy from that remote dim period of pre-history till now have been evident by different groups of people at different parts of the globe. It is evident that more than half of the world's modern drugs are of biological sources (Chakravorty *et al.,* 2011). Knowing the importance of it, tremendous works on plants used as medicinal therapy by different communities have been observed and a good collection and documentation of treasure of knowledge on it still go on. However, there is scanty information, poor research, and documentation on the using of animal and animal products for therapeutic treatments though it has been reported that of the 252 chemicals that have been selected by the WHO as essential to human health, 8.70 per cent come from animal sources (Chakravorty *et al.,* 2011). In this chapter, an attempt is being made to examine the uses different animal extracts for treatment purpose by the tribe of North East India.

Ethnozoological treatment among the tribes of North East India

Bear *(Selenarclos thibetanous)*. Among the Muklom Tangsa of New Thamlom village, Changlang district, Arunachal Pradesh '*Shap-lik*' (bear's gall bladder) is used as an ethnozoological therapy for curing malaria, high fever, and liver enlargement. Bear's gall bladder is dried over the hearth for at least 2-3 months. The local medicine man boils a small part of the gall bladder in water and feeds to the patient.

Among the Adis of Arunachal Pradesh, for treating dysentery, the gall bladder of bear locally known as *siitum* is dried over the hearth for months. The dried pieces of it are cooked and consumed by the patient. The Adis also use the teeth of a bear by making a necklace and wear to those persons who always afraid everything especially to *uyu* (evil spirits). The maternal aunt used to wear around the neck of her nephews who feel the fear of such spirits. A little quantity of bile of bear is taken with water for treating asthma among the Singphos of Arunachal Pradesh whereas the same procedure is used to cure blood dysentery among the Wanchos (Datta Chaudhuri, 2003). The Monpa of Arunachal Pradesh also use the bile and gallbladder of a bear, but not just for digestive disorders, but also for fighting malaria attacks (Solanki and Chutia, 2004). Among the Ao Naga of Nagaland, gall bladder of bear is applied externally over the wounds; with the help of penis of bear, it is easy to remove thorns in the flesh; hair is roasted, dissolved in water and orally administered for easy child delivery; fat is applied externally on the skin burn (Kakati and Doulo, 2002). The Ao Nagas boiled the bile of bear (*Shirem/Erem*) in water and drunk to cure malaria (Kakati *et al.,* 2006)

Among different groups Naga tribes in Nagaland, gall bladder, and bile duct extracts are used for relieving stomach disorders; fat is applied on joints to relieve rheumatic pain; touching testes facilitates delivery; flesh and penis are cooked and eaten to avoid general weakness (Jamir and Lal, 2005).

Python: Among the Muklom Tangsa, '*Pu-jong lik*' (Python's gall bladder) is no more available. It was believed to be a remedy for high fever and stomach enlargement. They believe that a sick person should be given a single dose only as more than one dose would make the sick person dies. They also make a paste from the python teeth *(Pu-jong pa)*. The tooth is scratch on a stone with water for a while, from which the paste is made and this paste is applied on the boiling part on the body. The tooth is very scarce and is used only in serious case.

Among the Adis, the fat of *Biirem Tabii* (python) is taken out from the snake and is stored in a container. It is used to massage the affected portion of the patient suffering from muscle pain or bone fracture among the Adis. The Nyishi and Galo use snakes in treating cattle that suffer from foot and mouth disease (Chakravartti *et al,* 2011). Among the Nagas of Nagaland, the bile duct of Python is used as an antidote against spider and snake bite; fat is applied to relieve body ache, rheumatic, pain and burn wounds (Jamir and Lal, 2005). The Mao Nagas burn the dried skin of Python and inhaled in order to ease child delivery.

Crab (*Cancer pararus):* Among the Mao Naga of Manipur, some herbs with the liquid extracted from crabs are mixed and given to drink to patients suffering from HIV-AIDS. What kind of herb is mixed with the crab was not revealed. The people also believed that eating of crab by cooking or frying cures small pox.

The whole body of crab is crushed into a paste and boiled in water to prepare a drink which helps different groups of Nagas in Nagaland in curing Jaundice and other liver disorders (Jamir and Lal, 2005)

Among the Chakhesang tribe of Nagaland, the whole body of crab is crushed, dissolved in waters and orally administered for treating arthritis; whole body is cooked, extract the soup and orally administered for treating cough and malaria; whole body is crashed, extract the liquid and 2-3 drops administered into the ear to cure earache; flesh is cooked and consumed to relieve stomach pain (Kakati and Doulo, 2002)

Egg of hen: Albumin of the egg is used for treating bone fracture among the Mao Naga tribe of Manipur. Albumin is put in the cotton to get wet and tied in the fracture part with a bamboo substitute as a bandage.

Among the Adis, raw eggs are directly consumed by the patient to cure soreness of throat. Only one raw egg is slowly consumed per day and continues until the sore heals.

By thoroughly mixing the yolk of the egg of black hen to honey and applying on the burnt surface, the Meiteis of Manipur used the mixture to cure fire burns.

Earthworm *(Pheritima* sps): The milky fluid produced by a big variety of earthworm is consumed by the patients particularly by children who suffer from ulcer and infection in the throat (who feel pain in swallowing food) among the Adis.

Earthworm is eaten raw to serve as an antidote in snake and spider bites by many Naga tribe in Nagaland (Jamir and Lal, 2005).The whole body of earthworm is crushed and locally applied on red eye to cure eye pain by the Chakhesang tribe of Nagaland (Kakati and Doulo, 2002).

Honey: Honey is given to patients who are suffering from a sore throat among the Adis; honey is regularly swallowed till the soreness is cured. They also use honey for curing cough. It is applied on the part of body injured by fire or steam burns. The Chakhesang tribe of Nagaland orally administered honey to cure a cough. They also locally applied honey over the wound to stop the loss of blood (Kakati and Doulo, 2002).

Hornbill *(Burcerotidae):* The fat of hornbill is massaged over fracture of bones, the dislocated part of bone or swelling among the Adis. Nyishis and Galos use the bird's cooked flesh specifically to ease the rheumatic pain (Chakravartti *et al*., 2011).

Eagle *(Aquila rapax):* Among the Muklom Tangsa, the beak of the eagle is scratched over a stone and makes a paste which is applied over boils and keeps for about 10 to 12 hours. Feather is locally applied over the wound (Kakati and Doulo, 2002). The fat of Eagle is applied for sprain, bone fracture and burn among the Chakhesang of Nagaland (Kakati *et al.,* 2006).

Among the Mishmis of Lohit district in Arunachal Pradesh, dried gall bladder of Eagle is mixed with water and taken twice a day during the late trimester of pregnancy for smooth delivery of baby (Sharma, 2007).

Mithun (*Bos frontalis*): Among the Adis, while breast feeding, if there is a pain in the breast of a lactating mother, a small part of roasted or smoked dried penis of Mithun is cooked and offered with warm water to the patient. Sometimes, the penis of *Mithun* is roasted and directly feed to the patient for the same problem. The eating of cooked penis to cure breast pain of a lactating mother is also found among the Ao Nagas of Nagaland who also uses the same for curing skin disease (Kakati *et al.,* 2006). Besides, different groups of Naga tribes use the same items for curing pain in the breast of lactating mother and skin disease of common people (Jamir and Lal, 2005). The Nysihis and the Galos of Arunachal Pradesh use the gall bladder of *Mithun* to cure dysentery, cough, and fever and also prescribe the testes of the bull to ease lactation problems of young mothers (Chakravorty *et al*., 2011).

Mongoose *(Herpestes* sp.*)*: An entire mongoose, eaten roasted or boiled, is believed to prevent many diseases by Arunachal tribes (Chakravorty *et al.,* 2011).The penis of mongoose is properly cooked and orally taken to cure male impotency among the Ao Naga of Nagaland

(Kakati *et al.,* 2006). Among the Adis, the soup of mongoose is given to patients to cure T.B.

Tiger (*Panthera tigris tigris*): Many parts of tiger such as bones, claws, and whiskers are used in making charms, which are thought to bring strength and vigour to the wearer and frighten the enemy. In an earlier time, among the Meiteis of Manipur, tiger milk is given to male children who are weak and inactive so that they become active, brave and strong like a tiger. The Nyishi tribe used the bone of tiger for treating jaundice whereas the Monpa tribe used dried tiger bone powder to ease rheumatic pains (Solanki and Chutia, 2004); the Adis use the fat of tiger to relieve from joint and muscle pains; the fat is applied for relieving body ache and rheumatic pain and the milk cures cataract and night blindness as is believed by different Naga groups of Nagaland (Jamir and Lal, 2005).

Jackal/Fox (*Canis* sps.): The flesh of the fox, given to Nyishi and Galo children, is believed to turn the children into cunning adults, but the flesh is also used as a tuberculosis remedy amongst the Nyishi; among the Adis, the boiled flesh is boiled is given to cure fever and malaria.

Different groups of Nagas of Nagaland believed that the eating of the flesh of Jackal/Fox (*Canis* sps.) helps in relieving cholera, asthma, tuberculosis and chest pain whereas the fat of the animal is applied to relieve and cure bodyache, rheumatic pain and skin diseases of (Jamir and Lal, 2005). Among the Ao Nagas of Nagaland, urine of flying fox is soaked in rice, dried and taken to cure kidney stones (Kakati *et al.,* 2006).

Porcupine (*Hystrix* sps): Nyishis and Galos treat individuals suffering from tuberculosis by eating the flesh of porcupine. Among the Adis, the stomach of Indian porcupine is boiled with water and given to patients to cure asthma, dysentery, gastric pain, diarrhea and joint pain and is found to be effective (Sharma, 2007). The smoked dried gall bladder is boiled with water and given to patients to cure of dysentery and fever (Sharma, 2007). The Wanchos dried the stomach of porcupine and is boiled and have it to cure blood dysentery (Datta Chaudhuri, 2003).

The Khamptis of Arunachal Pradesh treats asthma in which a patient has respiratory trouble, the intestine of the porcupine is burnt in fire and the ash is dissolved in a glass of water. Before taking a meal, the water is drunk three times a day (Bhowmick, 2003). The Digaru Mishmis burnt the spikes of porcupine and a pinch of ash is orally taken to cure dysentery and fever (Bhowmick, 2003).

Naga tribes of Nagaland apply the fat of porcupine to get relief from body ache, rheumatic pain, burn-wounds and rapid healing of fractured bones; by drinking the water which was dipped overnight with the dried stomach, they attempt to cure cholera, dysentery and stomach disorders (Jamir and Lal, 2005).

The Chakhesang tribe of Nagaland roast the porcupine spine and orally administered to reduce bone fracture and pain; small intestine is boiled with water and orally administered to cure gastritis; dried and powdered the stomach, boiled and orally administered to cure fever (Kakati and Doulo, 2002).The Ao Nagas of Nagaland soaked the bile of porcupine in rice, then make it dry and taken for treating dysentery (Kakati *et al.,* 2006).

Deer: The granules of the musk of musk deer are taken orally by the Digaru Mishmis of Arunachal Pradesh to cure pain in the stomach and toothache. They also use a common deer's skin by burning and inhaling the gas to cure stomach pain (Bhowmick, 2003). Among the Adis, the musk gland situated beneath the skin of the abdomen of the male deer is used as medicine to cure fever, malaria and stomach pains (Sharma, 2007). Crushed antlers of the Sambar deer are used by the Galo for bursting open boils.

Musk deer *(Maschus* sp.*)* flesh is used for enhancing body immunity and resistance to malaria by the Ao Naga of Nagaland, and the Mompa of Arunachal Pradesh (Chakravartti *et al.,* 2011).

Many different tribal Naga groups of Nagaland powdered the bones of deer and suspended in water and drop the water into the affected areas such as earache, chest pain, rheumatic pain, and fever; the soup made from the leg of deer is believed to ease delivery and the fat is used for treating burns and piles (Jamir and Lal, 2005). The Chakhesang tribe of Nagaland also used the urine of musk deer as ear drop to cure ear swelling and pain; they also orally taken the blood of the deer to cure stomach pain and anaemia (Kakati and Doulo, 2002).

Tortoise (*Testudo* sp.): The Muklom Tangsa of Arunachal Pradesh make a paste of the hard shell of a tortoise by scratching over a stone and applied on the skin infected with ring worms or by mud. They first clean the infected area with salt. The Ao Naga tribe of Nagaland cooks and eats the flesh of tortoise to cure piles and skin disease (Kakati *et al.,* 2006).

Conclusion

Plants and animals are unavoidable resources for human survival and use as food. The extracts from plants and animals have been utilising for treatment purpose for different health problems from time immemorial. People of North East India, because of their rich biodiversity, vast coverage of land by forest and having many ethnic compositions tap these resources in one way or another. Using of these floral and faunal products for health and treatment is one such indigenous knowledge of these people.

The use of different ethnozoological products by the people may have scientific validation or just the otherwise. It may be conjectured that our ancestors when they faced health and health-related problems; they might have attempted different means of solving the problems. In order to poise their distress mind, they practice magico-religious procedures of treatment. Sometimes, when magic and prayer failed, they might have started looking for the other option i.e. science. Deliberately or accidentally, some herbs or products of animals might have given relief and easiness for their particular health problems. Their curiosity made them wiser and from such experience and experiments by trial and error, they found the utility of using such floral and faunal products. However, it is a challenge to the modern researchers to validate the effects of such ethnomedicines. Some researchers validated many plants and animals. For instance, one of the widely used plants for abortion and widely available in North East India including Assam, *Trichosanthes palmata*, is found to have properties of anti-fertility when experimented in the laboratory in rats (Sharma, 2007). On the value of medicinal property of animal product, Chakravorty *et al.*, (2011) say "Although traditional treatments, making use of animals or animal parts, have often been considered mere superstition, their persistence over hundreds or even thousands of years ought to be sufficient incentive to probe whether or not they are effective. And sure enough, the potency of at least some traditional medicines based on animals cannot be denied, since numerous such medicines have been methodically tested by pharmaceutical companies and turned into sources of drugs, which are now part of the armament of the modern healer (Chakravorty *et al.*, 2011). For instance, peptides extracted from scraped secretions of *Phyllomedusa bicolor* (amphibians) found in Amazon basin, are used in the treatment of depression, stroke, seizures and cognitive loss in ailments such as Alzheimer's disease (Amato, 1992; Daly *et al.,* 1992). Early muscle relaxants were obtained from so-called poison arrow frogs, containing curare, a compound also used in psychiatric treatments. The deer velvet extract pantocrin is nowadays marketed as a powerful antioxidant with anti-stress and immune-modulatory activity for use in humans and animals (Je *et al*., 2010)". However, many of the ethnomedicinal plants and animals are not necessarily inherently useful for treatment. If we examine in the present discussion, it is vividly seen that the using of certain animal products to cure certain health problems are based on the simple logic of pre-literate people without having any scientific reasons. For instance, 'the wings of fire fly are removed and are inserted in to the banana and given to eat the patients suffering from night blindness among the Adis, the wearing of bear or tiger teeth to persons who are mentally weak and depress among the Adis, the flesh of the fox, given to Nyishi and Galo children, is supposed to turn the children into cunning, mongoose penis is used to treat impotence amongst the Ao Naga and so on. If the chemical composition of the product has no positive reaction to the biology of the patient and yet if the product is still functional, then perhaps, it may have some psychosomatic reaction like what so called 'placebo effect'.

Another dimension that we can look into is that the modern allopathic system cannot deliver all the health needs of the people. For one reason, accessibility to such modern health delivery system is not for all; the other reason is that many people still believe their deep-rooted cultural beliefs and practices and they utilise it. Even many learned people who have awareness and accessibility to modern medical amenities still embrace their traditional medicine or both, 'medical pluralism'. Therefore, what is required is a refining of the system for the practical utility to the people. Giving training on the crude system of practices of traditional medicine of the local medicine-men with scientific method and technique of health and hygiene shall benefit to people particularly to those who do not have the accessibility of modern health delivery system.

Another dimension is the role to play in keeping conservation of biodiversity. Unnecessarily killing of endangered species of animals and medicinal plants for profit motif shall be checked. Rather scope for planting medicinal plants and rearing of animals for catering to the needs of pharmaceutical demands with necessary financial aid and training and other resources shall solve at least some problems of unemployment.

References

Amato, I, 1992. 'From hunter magic, a pharmacopeia?' *Science,* 258, 5086: 1306.

Bhowmick, DC, 2003a. 'Indigenous health practices among the Digaru Mishmis of Arunachal Pradesh'. *Journal of Anthropological Survey of India*, 52,4: 1-8.

Bhowmick, DC, 2003b. 'Indigenous health practices among the Khamptis of Arunachal Pradesh'. *Journal of Anthropological Survey of India*, 52: 57-66.

Chakravorty, J; VB Meyer-Rochow and S Ghosh. 2011, 'Vertebrates used for medicinal purposes by members of the Nyishi and Galo tribes in Arunachal Pradesh, North East India'. *Ethnobiol Ethnomed.* 7: 13.

Daly, JW; J. Caceres; RW Moni; F. Gusovsky; M. Moos; Jr.KB Seamon; K. Milton; and CW Myers. 1992. 'Frog secretion and hunting magic in the upper Amazon: Identification of a peptide that interacts with an adenosine receptor'. *Proc. Natl. Acad. Sci.* 89: 10960-10963.

Datta Chaudhuri, SS, 2003a. 'Indigenous health practices system among the Singphos of Arunachal Pradesh', *Journal of Anthropological Survey of India*: 52: 49-55.

Datta Chaudhuri, SS, 2003b. 'Traditional way of healing system among the Wancho of Tirap district, Arunachal Pradesh', *Journal of Anthropological Survey of India*: 52.

Jamir, NS and P Lal 2005. 'Ethnozoological practices among Naga tribes'. *Indian Journal of Traditional Knowledge,* 4, 1: 100-104.

Je, JY; PJ. Park; EK Kim; HA. Kim; DH. Lim; BT Jeon; and CB Ahn. 2010. 'Composition of biologically active substance and antioxidant activity of New Zealand Deer Velvet Antler extracts'. *Korean J. Food Sci. Anti. Resour.* 30: 20-27.

Kakati, LN. and V Doulo, 2002. 'Indigenous knowledge system of zoo-therapeutic use by Chakhesang tribe of Nagaland, India'. *Journal of Human Ecology,* 13, 6: 419-423.

Kakati, LN.; Bendang Ao and V Doulo, 2006. 'Indigenous knowledge of the zoo-therapeutic use of vertebrate origin by the Ao tribe of Nagaland'. *Journal of Human Ecology*, 19, 3: 163-167.

Padmanabham, P and KA Sujana.2008. 'Animal products in traditional medicine from Attappady hills of Western Ghats'. *Indian Journal of Traditional Knowledge*. 7:326–329.

Sarma, HN, 2007. *Traditional Medicine of Arunachal Pradesh - Practice and Prospect*, Guwahati; Grantha Peeth.

Solanki, GS, and P Chutia. 2004. 'Ethnozoological and socio-cultural aspects of Monpas of Arunachal Pradesh'. *Journal of Human Ecology*. 15, 4:251–254.

Chapter - 4

Indigenous Knowledge Base for Development of Green Manufacturing and Cost Effective Healthcare

—Nikhil K Sachan, Seema Pushkar, and S.K. Ghosh

Introduction

Sophisticated knowledge of the natural world is not confined to science. Human societies all across the globe have developed rich sets of experiences and explanations relating to the environments they live in. These 'other knowledge systems' are today often referred to as traditional ecological knowledge or indigenous or local knowledge. They encompass the sophisticated arrays of information, understandings, and interpretations that guide human societies around the globe in their innumerable interactions with the natural milieu: in agriculture and animal husbandry; hunting, fishing and gathering; struggles against disease and injury; naming and explanation of natural phenomena; and strategies to cope with fluctuating environments (Nakashima *et al.*, 2000). An indigenous person is defined largely through self-identification as indigenous or tribal. Indigenous communities, peoples, and nations are those which have a historical continuity with pre-invasion and pre-colonial societies that developed on their territories; consider themselves distinct from other sectors of societies now prevailing in those territories, or parts of them. They form at present non-dominant sectors of society and are determined to preserve, develop, and transmit to future generations their ancestral territories, and their ethnic identity, as the basis of their continued existences as peoples, in accordance with their own cultural patterns, social institutions and legal systems (Martinez Cobo, 1986; UNDP, 2003). In other words, indigenous people were original inhabitants of a specific location (Struthers *et al.*, 2004). Indigenous people have a broad knowledge of how to live sustainably. However, formal education systems have disrupted the practical everyday life aspects of indigenous knowledge and ways of learning, replacing them with abstract knowledge and academic ways of learning. The Indigenous Knowledge (IK), therefore, is the local knowledge that is unique to a culture or society it may also call as 'local knowledge', 'folk knowledge', 'people's knowledge', 'traditional wisdom' or 'traditional science' etc. This knowledge is carried forward from generation to generation, usually by words of mouth and cultural rituals, and has been the basis for agriculture, food preparation, healthcare, education, conservation and the wide range of other activities that sustain societies in many parts of the world. IK is stored in peoples' memories and activities and is expressed in stories, songs, folklore, proverbs, dances, myths, cultural values, beliefs, rituals, community laws, local language and taxonomy, agricultural practices, equipment, materials, plant species, and animal breeds. IK is shared and communicated orally, by specific example, and through culture (Grenier, 1998). IK is usually collective knowledge; sometimes, due to parallel development or due to the exchange of knowledge, communities with similar ecosystems, culture or problems can have the same or similar IK which, in turn, is or is not, expressed in a similar fashion (Maden *et al.,* 1994).

Today the pharmaceutical industry is a powerhouse performer; it is the notable sign of globalisation and capitalism that there is a high degree of competition of in terms of money and time in the field of drugs and pharmaceutical research (Sachan, 2010). The major focus of the research carried out on the value of genetic resources has been on their use in the pharmaceutical and agricultural industries, which use genetic diversity as a source of information in their development of new products. Economists have long analysed the research and development process as one of information utilisation, application, and diffusion. The concept of research and development is usually presented as a production process itself dependent upon a stock of "information" for its generation of useful innovations (water insoluble drug paper). Practiced traditions can offer a more holistic approach to drug design and myriad possible targets for scientific analysis toward the drug development may it be the newer constituent for a therapeutic purpose or otherwise materials for drug product development enhancing the performance and effectiveness of drugs in the body and/or improving patient compliance. Traditional knowledge can serve as a powerful search engine, which will greatly facilitate intentionally, focused and safe natural product drug discovery and help to rediscover the drug discovery process. By looking at the historical trends in drug and medical developments, it is possible to understand how current drug development will benefit from this partnership. The input of traditional knowledge regarding medicinal importance of certain plants works as a shortcut and hasten the process of screening simultaneously this also reduce the cost of drug development process.

Drug Delivery Enhanced Products in Healthcare Market

Drug Discovery in the current scenario has become unproductive to the point where the economic future of the industry is questionable. To push into the future, the R and D thrust in the pharmaceutical sector needs to be focused on the development of new drugs, innovative processes for known drugs and development of plant-based drugs through investigation of leads from the traditional systems of medicine. The Drug delivery, in fact, is highly innovative in terms of materials to assist delivery, excipients, and technology which allow the fast or slow release of drugs (Sachan *et al.,* 2010). All therapeutic products, including therapeutic products for human and veterinary use, include excipients - indeed, the total amount of excipients frequently used is greater than the amount of the active drug substance(s) in a dosage form. Therefore the pharmaceutical excipients are having a key role to play in the formulation of drug delivery systems. They can affect the overall efficacy and cost effectiveness of the dosage form (Sachan and Bhattacharya, 2006). Formulators apply a practical understanding of pharmaceutical excipients to develop optimal, robust formulations and the appropriate manufacturing processes. During the past few years, the industry has come to understand better, the excipient functionality and variability as well as excipients' role in the drug product supply chain (Drakulich, 2010). As any formulation which is having a different composition is considered to be new drug so the existing patent regime will not be applicable to them. So if a new excipient with similar functionality can be incorporated into a patented formulation then such a modified drug product can be manufactured being out of patent coverage or, otherwise the same can be patented separately by the same or another pharmaceutical firm in view of extension of patent/re-patentability or getting out of paying royalty (Sachan, 2009). Therefore presently in highly competitive and increasingly global pharmaceutical market, when there is a mounting pressure on the research and development (R and D), to shorten development time and get products to the market faster with a cost effective formulation, new pharmaceutical excipients appears to be the master key at techno scientific level for financial planning and performance of pharmaceutical industries in developing countries. The substantial amount of research have been poured in the field of formulation excipients, exploring these supposedly inert materials for their better compatibility with active ingredients, improved stability, cost effectiveness and associated desirable features demanded by the product for handling, aesthetic acceptance, and aid in the delivery of drug (Sachan and Singh, 2006).

The better excipients have been continuously in demand to overcome the cost barriers, for better pharmacokinetic profile and to by-pass the patent barriers in the manufacture of certain products by pharmaceutical industries which could have otherwise been protected by patents and require regulatory processes for grant of permission to manufacture from innovator and are costly affairs (Shangraw and Demarest, 1993; Frost and Sullivan, 2005). With more than 50 patents expired recently and several other in the queue, which includes a number of blockbuster drugs, pharmaceutical companies are recognising drug delivery technology, which is based on the use of polymer, as a powerful strategic marketing tool to differentiate products. This enables them to extend product life cycle and remains competitive in the marketplace (Oelkers and Elsey, 2003; Shenoy, 2003; Kashyap *et al.,* 2004). By infusing drugs with new and innovative therapeutic benefits, drug delivery systems extend products profitable life cycle, giving pharmaceutical companies competitive and financial advantages and providing patients with improved medications.

On the business end, for the pharmaceutical industry, extended release oral dosage forms provide multiple commercial benefits including patient-related factors like improved compliance and better therapeutic outcomes, as well as the new formulations can also extend market exclusivity. As a matter of time, excipient research has proven a versatile tool for growth and survival of pharmaceutical firms with a huge impact on the business through drug delivery enhanced and/or enabled products [DDEP]. The companies can enjoy an extension of the market exclusivity or the patent by reformulation with new excipients of their products for those the patents that are about to expire. Moreover, the functionally equivalent DDEPs have also become a major area of research for the industries towards getting market exclusivity and to manufacture a product which got patented by incorporating the new excipients in the formulation. These functionally equivalent DDEPs incorporate the same actives but use non-patent infringing drug delivery systems. In the marketplace, this means the DDEPs enjoy, market exclusivity independently from generics or any patent protection existing for pharmaceutical actives (API). It is interesting to speculate that the development and approval time for oral DDEPs are much shorter and market exclusivity with regard to generic products is approved solely on the basis of bioequivalence data (Bossart, 2010).

Concept and Methodology

The Assam *Bora* rice is glutinous rice cultivated in Assam region. The starch is known as a glutinous or waxy starch when it contains very low amylase, generally less than three per cent by weight. The present investigation was undertaken to explore the pharmaceutical utility of Assam *Bora* rice, as in North East India this particular variety of rice is special ethnic significance. It is believed that the famous Shiva temple located at Sibsagar, Assam was constructed by joining the bricks using this rice paste along with duck egg as cement. The *Bora* rice is also used in the preparation of '*Peetha*'–an ethnic festive dish of Assam. There also this rice serves as a major binder, it indicates the adhesive behaviour of rice starch. Based on the information gained from traditional cultivators and scientists from Assam Agriculture University (Pathak *et al.,* 1995), it was affirmed that the *Bora* rice is sticky rice having binding properties and that is because of its low amylase content and is composed of almost entirely with amylopectin. The amylase is a linear polymer account mainly for the disintegration property of starch; on the other hand, amylopectin is a highly branched polymer probably responsible for retarding the degradation and release of entrapped chemical from the matrix (Peerapattana *et al.,* 2004). Keeping in view of these facts this holistically inspired study was undertaken with scientific guidance from International Pharmaceutical Excipient Council to explore this potential material for use in drug delivery as an economic biocompatible polymer for modulated release systems.

In contemporary scenario, to improvise research attempts and shorten the time in discovery and development it is customary to explore and interpret the cultural and ethnic knowledge heritage. The holistic information coined in our cultures and customs have a scientific basis and many times this may seek a new source of inspiration with the research started on plant-based drugs as a clue or short-cut of much rigorous and in-depth multiple trial experimentation. The scientific method called "positivism" gains significance in this context. In this connection, using *Bora* rice as a pharmaceutical excipient is potentially interesting as it is a common foodstuff and can be classified as 'GRAS' (Generally regarded as safe), which is necessary for any new excipient to be used in food or pharmaceuticals for the regulatory purpose (Rados, 2004). It is a high-cost affair and because of this, there are only a handful of substances from in numerous researched materials could be scaled up for industrial use. The natural materials have been extensively used in the field of drug delivery also because they are readily available, cost-effective, eco-friendly, capable of chemical modifications, potentially degradable and compatible due to their natural origin. In addition, this can be a potential marketing tool in the 'herbal boom worldwide', the present day consumer looks for the natural ingredients in the food drug and cosmetics as they believe that anything natural will be safer and devoid of side effects as compared to their synthetic counterparts.

Based on the above holistic, ethnobotanical and phytochemical facts, the *Bora* rice was investigated for its pharmaceutical utility as drug delivery excipient wherein the micro particulate drug delivery systems were formulated using natural polymeric backbone using this rice with and without the combination of another biopolymeric material. The prepared micro carriers were subjected to evaluation under the light of pharmaceutical principles, compendia standards and regulatory guidelines for new drug products. The *Bora* rice was procured from the local market of Dibrugarh Assam. Drug samples were obtained as gift sample from industrial sources. All other chemicals used were the analytical grade laboratory reagents and were used as such without further testing. The starch material was isolated through an established alkaline extraction method and product so obtained was characterised for pharmacy technical fitness for its use in pharmaceutical purpose (Kumar, 2011).

This rice was then gelatinised and blended with the drug to formulate inappropriate manner (Sachan and Bhattacharya, 2009) and tested using instrumental techniques for obtaining information in support of claimed usage. Most important, the stickiness of rice, its swelling behaviour, the capacity to hold drug and release it inside the body in a manner as intended for the cure of diseases and improving patient compliance was particularly tested. The results were statistically validated for reproducibility and interdependence of various factors.

Results and Discussions

The isolated rice starch was found to be composed of almost 100.0 per cent (>99 per cent) of amylopectin and only traces of amylase, starch lipids, protein and fibers. Further quadruplicate testing on three samples of whole grain *Bora* rice powder showed on average amylase content as 0.257 per cent. The highest amylase content tested in one sample was found to be 0.715 percent. The total amylopectin content was more than 98.0 per cent of total dry weight. Average particle size in rice powder was found to be 21.75 μm; however, most of the particles lie between 8-12 μm.

Pharmacotechnical characterisation of powdered *Bora* rice revealed the poor flow property of the powder. It also pointed to low water solubility and thus the need of thermal modification of sample for incorporation of drugs (Table 4.1). The thermal gelatinisation of rice could be done by heating above its glass transition temperature (Tg) which was found to be 65°C in DSC analysis. The thermal analysis also revealed the semi-crystalline nature of glutinous rice starch undergoing two stages of melting

Table 4.1: Pharmacotechnical Properties of Bora rice

Cold water solubility (g/dm^3) ± SD	1.01 ± 0.08
Average particle size (μm) ± SD	21.75 ± 12.65
True density (g/cm^3) ± SD	1.74 ± 0.03
Bulk density (g/cm^3) ± SD	0.31 ± 0.06
Tapped density (g/cm^3) ± SD	0.46 ± 0.01
Carr's Compressibility Index (%) ± SD	31.93 ± 2.88
Hausner's Ratio ± SD	1.47 ± 0.06
Angle of repose (θ) ± SD	40.31 ± 1.52

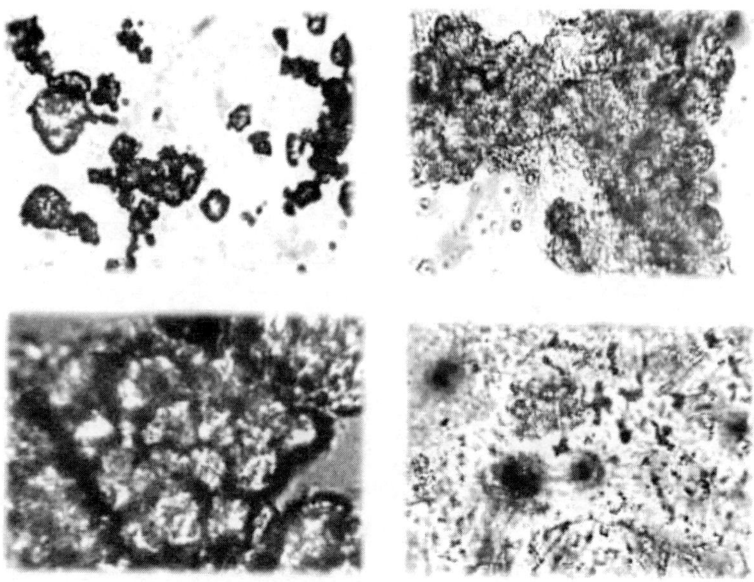

Figure 4.1: Photomicrographs of Thermal Gelation of Bora Rice

for intervening amorphous and crystalline structures. Structural inference, about *Bora* rice granules, from DSC and X-ray diffraction, provides an explanation for the possible functionality of biopolymeric backbone for modulated release of medicament discussed widely in the thesis. Microscopic investigations of gelatinizing *Bora* rice granules supported the findings of DSC and reflect the various stages in gelatinisation to be completed before the drug is added for incorporation as guest molecule by retrogradation (Fig. 4.1).

Micro-carriers with Assam *Bora* rice backbone have shown excellent DEE with Ibuprofen and Flurbiprofen but it has shown comparatively poor drug entrapment efficiency for highly water soluble drug Metformin hydrochloride, for which the modified ionic gelation method, produced microcarriers with improved drug entrapment up to 81 per cent. The average drug entrapment efficiency of micro carriers prepared by emulsion polymerisation was 91.06±1.03 per cent, for epichlorohydrin cross-linked micro-carriers 84.90±1.44 and 89.03±1.12 for TMP cross-linked micro-carriers. Water sorption studies revealed the variable swelling of micro carriers in different pH environments which provide a major correlation for the drug release behavior which may be attributed for the chain relaxation due to swelling of the backbone. Prepared micro-carriers by ionic gelation were sufficiently similar irrespective of the drug used. The percentage water sorption by weight (swelling ratio) of carriers in the different medium after 48 hours was calculated for the micro-carriers prepared (Fig. 4.2).

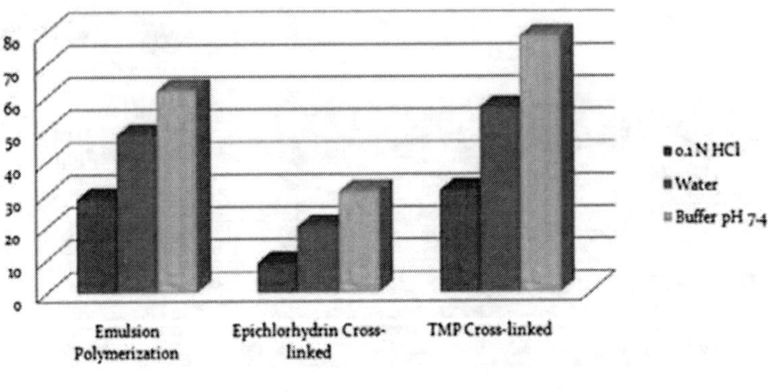

Figure 4.2: Water Sorption by Drug Loaded Bora Rice Microcarriers.

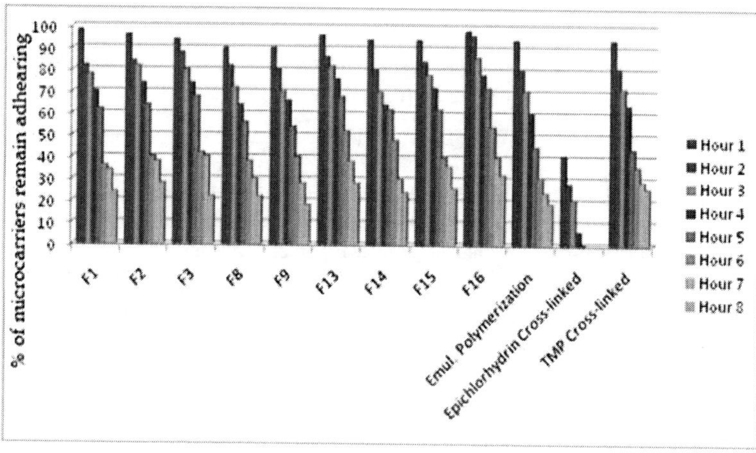

Figure 4.3: Wash-off Profile of Micro-carriers Showing Mucoadhesion.

The wash-off profile of prepared micro-carriers reflects the excellent mucoadhesive *in vitro* when compared to the non-mucoadhesive material (Fig. 4.3). Epichlorohydrin treatment significantly reduced the mucoadhesive of the polymer backbone, therefore, it may not be considered suitable as such for the preparation of drug loaded micro-carriers where mucoadhesive is desired. This can be due to the uncontrolled blocking of free hydroxyl groups which are held responsible for attachment with mucosa. TMP cross-linked micro-carriers showed better mucoadhesive than those prepared by emulsion polymerisation.

The mucoadhesive of the micro-carriers was also dependent on the medium. Buffer medium causes gelation of the micro-carriers and erosion of micro-carriers.

Conclusions

In conclusion, the pharmaceutical assessment of *Bora* rice and fabricated micro devices revealed the potential of *Bora* rice based biopolymeric backbone in drug delivery and it is worth full to mention here that the use of proposed biopolymer has shown a good degree of binding property in reformulation study, as claimed holistically being used in the holy Shivsagar temple. The *Bora* rice is having good mucoadhesion and capable of prolonged drug release with potential for further modifications in prepared micro devices to be used in the controlled drug delivery.

References

Bossart, J. 1010. 'Oral drug delivery: The numbers behind the business', in *Oral Drug Delivery and Advanced Excipients,* pp. 04-06, East Sussex, U.K.; Frederick Furness Publishing. Available through: www. Ondrugdelivery. com.

Drakulich, A. 2010. 'Excipients steps into the spotlight'. *Pharmaceutical Technology.* 6, 34: 34-42.

Frost, LA, and DL Sullivan. 2005. 'Strategic analysis of pharmaceutical excipients market in Europe'. May 12, 2005. http://www.marketresearch.com/Frost-Sullivan-v383/Strategic-Pharmaceutical-Excipients-Europe-1117743/(accessed March 20, 2013).

Grenier, L.1998. *Working with Indigenous Knowledge: A Guide for Researchers.* Ottawa, Canada; International Development Research Centre. http://himalaya.socanth.cam.ac.uk/collections/rarebooks/downloads/Maden_Indigenous_Knowledge.pdf (accessed March 17, 2013).

Kashyap, N; S Modi; JP Jain; I Bala; S Hariharan; R Bhardwaj; D Singh; R Mahajan; N Kumar, and MNV Ravi Kumar, 2004. 'Polymers for advanced drug delivery'. *CRIPS*, 5, 3: 7-12.

Maden, K; R Kongren and TM Limbu.1994. 'Digital Himalaya'. In Alan Macfarlane and Mark Turin (Eds): *Documentation of Indigenous Knowledge, Skill and Practices of Kirata. Nationalities with Special Focus on Biological Resources.* The University of Cambridge.

Martinez Cobo Jr.1986. *Study of the Problem of Discrimination against Indigenous Populations* Final Report, Geneva, Switzerland; United Nations Economic and Social Council.

Nakashima, D; L Prott and P Bridgewater. 2000. 'Tapping into the World's Wisdom'. *UNESCO Sources*, (English edition): pp 11-12.

Oelkers, G and B Elsey. 2003. 'The economic effects on the international pharmaceutical industry of the trade-related aspects of intellectual property rights (Trips) agreement on patent protection in Indonesia'. *ABAC Journal*, 23,1: 34-60.

Pathak, PK; T Ahmed; KK Sharma and AK Pathak, 1995. 'High yielding glutinous rice varieties in Assam'. *Oryza*, 32: 48–50.

Peerapattana, J; A Tattawasart and V Srijesdaruk, 2004. 'Modified glutinous starch as a hydrophilic matrix substance'. *Thai J. Pharm. Sci,* 28, 1-2: 57-72.

Rados, C, 2004. 'GRAS: Time-tested, and trusted, food ingredients'. *FDA Consumer Magazine 2004* (March - April). Available through: http://www.fda.gov /FDIC/ features/ 2004/204_gras.html (accessed on: Aug 28, 2005)

Sachan, NK and A Bhattacharya. 2009. 'Modelling and characterisation of drug release from glutinous rice starch based hydrogel beads for controlled drug delivery'. *International Journal of Health Research,* 2,1: 113-119.

Sachan, NK and A Bhattacharya. 2006. 'Evaluation of Assam Bora rice starch as a possible natural mucoadhesive polymer in the formulation of micro particulate controlled drug delivery systems'. *Journal of Assam Science Society*, 46: 34-41.

Sachan, NK and D Singh. 2006. 'Evaluation of dried pulp from fruits of *Carica papaya* as a disintegrating agent in the metformin hydrochloride dispersible tablets'. *Journal of Assam Science Society* 46, 2: 20 - 22.

Sachan, NK 2009. 'Regulatory interventions of new drug approval and conduct of clinical trials in India'. *Pharma News Letter*, September issue: 05-07.

Sachan, NK 2010. 'Contribution of Indian traditional and holistic medicine to new drug development', In Arvind Kumar and Govind Das (Eds): *Biodiversity, Biotechnology and Traditional Knowledge: Understanding Intellectual Property Rights*, pp. 175 - 190. New Delhi; Narosa Publishing House.

Sachan, NK; SK Ghosh and S Pushkar. 2010. 'Science of polymeric plant based excipients in pharmaceutical drug delivery systems'. *Global Perspectives of Biological Research in the Present Scenario.* pp. 135-150.

Sachan, NK 2011. *Fabrication and Biopharmaceutical Characterisation of Microparticulate Controlled drug Delivery System Composed of Assam Bora Rice as Possible Mucoadhesive Backbone.* Unpublished Ph.D. Thesis, Dibrugarh University, Dibrugarh, Assam.

Shangraw, RR and DA Demarest. 1993. 'Survey of current practices in the formulation and manufacture of tablets and capsules'. *Pharmaceutical Technology,* 17: 32-44.

Shenoy, PKR 2003. 'A strategic insight'. In *Pharma Technology/Express Pharma Pulse* Special Feature | May 29, 2003: pp. 16-18. Available through: *www.expresspharmaonline.com/pharmatech.pdf (accessed on May 29, 2011).*

Struthers, R; S Valerie; S Eschiti and B Patchell, 2004. 'Traditional indigenous healing: Part I'. *Complementary Therapies in Nursing and Midwifery* 10: 140–149.

UNDP. 2003. *United Nations Development Programme: About Indigenous People-Definition.* 2003.http://www.undp.org/csopp/CSO/NewFiles/ipaboutdef.html (accessed December 26, 2003).

Chapter - 5

Ethnomedicinal Practices among the Karbis of Assam

—Melody Seb Rengma, Sar-Im Tisso, and Longkiri Timung

Introduction

The Study of Indigenous medicine or medicinal features generally referred to as 'ethnomedicine'. Ethnomedicine has been recognised as an important field of Anthropological research. The study of ethnomedicine primarily aims at exploring various aspects of diseases, magico-religious and other therapies, indigenous preventive measure, the role of folk medicine men etc. It also includes the socio-cultural dimensions of indigenous medicinal features and the relationship between medical phenomenon and socio-cultural settings. According to Foster and Anderson (1978), "Ethnomedicine denotes the totality of health knowledge, value, beliefs, skills, and practices of indigenous people including all clinical and non-clinical activities that relate to their needs". World Health Organisation (WHO) estimated that not less than 2,02,000 species of plants are used as medicinal plants (c.f Gupta and Chadha,1995), and 80.00 per cent of the world population relies largely on or solely on traditional remedies for healthcare (c.f Bannerman,1982). According to the data released by WHO (2003), Ethnomedicine has maintained its popularity in all regions of developing the world and its use is expanding in the industrialised world. Choi *et al* (2013) study refer that the use of bamboo leaves (*Phyllostachys* pubescent Mazel ex J. Houz (*Poaceae*) have a long history of food and medical applications in Asia including Japan and Korea. They have been used as a traditional medicine for centuries. Some of the studies done in India include studies on ethnomedicinal plants conserved by Garasia tribes (Meena and Jadav, 2010), Srinivasa (2010) works on ethnomedical practices among the Jenu Kuruba of Karnataka. Jeetendra and Kumar (2012) recorded ethnomedicinal plants used by tribal communities for the treatment of snakebite in West Nimar, M.P. Northeastern part of India is also not an exception. A number of studies on Ethnomedicine have been undertaken by different workers from different states of Northeast India. It has also been reported that Boro tribes of Assam used various medicinal plants for family planning and birth control (Tiwari *et al.*, 1979). Some other uses of medicinal plants by Boro tribes also been reported from Assam (Baruah and Sharma, 1984). The Mao Naga of Manipur practices folk medicines to take care of their health and related problems primarily from the plant resources available within and the vicinity of their environment (Lokho, 2012). The people of the North-eastern region of India use at least 65 plants belonging to 38 families to treat malaria. Different plant parts such as the leaf, root, bark and fruit and in some cases the whole plant were used for making the herbal preparations (Bora *et al.,* 2007). Ethno-Medicinal Practices among the Sonowal Kacharis was further done by (Das *et al.,* 2008). Very few studies on indigenous health practices have so far been done among Karbi people from Karbi Anglong district of Assam. Talukdar (2002) conducted a study on beliefs and practices regarding disease and treatment among the Karbis of Assam. There are varieties species of wild vegetables and varieties species of medicinal plants used by the Karbi people. They consume wild vegetables which have a high medicinal value and possess the knowledge of curing disease and ailments by using medicinal plants. They also practice magico-religious and perform rituals in order to cure disease however the present study put more emphasis on medicinal plants and wild vegetables that are incorporated by the people of Karbis. Therefore the present study aims to find out and document their various aspects of health and treatment by using different herbs and medicinal plant among the Karbi people of Karbi Anglong district of Assam.

The present study has been focused on the following two aspects; (i) to document the medicinal plants used by the Karbis, and (ii) to know their various ways of treatment.

Study Population

Karbi Anglong District is situated in the central part of Assam. The district is situated between 25°33' N to 26°35' N Latitude and 92°10' to 93°50' E Longitude with a total geographical area of 10,434 sq. km. According to 2011 census, the district has a total population of 965,280 of which male and female populations were 493,482 and 471,798 respectively. The district could be broadly divided into two physiographic unit's *viz.*

hills and plains. However, 85 per cent of the district was covered by hills. Moist-semi evergreen forest, Moist Mixed Deciduous Forest, Riverrain type, and miscellaneous type with scattered pure or mixed patches of bamboos are the forest types of the district.

The Karbis are the dominant tribal group in the district. Besides a number of other tribal groups like Bodos, Kukis, Dimasas, Hmars, Garos, Rengma Nagas, Tiwas, Maan and a large number of non-tribals also found in the district. Ethnically the Karbis belong to Mongoloid group and speak the languages of Tibeto-Burman group. The term "Karbi" is derived from the word *"Thekar Kibi"* meaning offering of household deities before eating or drinking either in private or in a social occasion. The Karbis have five clans called "*nok-hum*". These are Ejang (Enghi), Tunjang (Timung), Kronjang (Teron), Lijang (Engti) and Hangjang (Terang). These clans are completely exogamous and marriage between a boy and a girl belonging to the same clan can never take place since the children of the same clan are considered as brother and sister. Violation of this customary law obviously leads to the excommunication of the couple involved.

The present study was done on the Karbi of Ram Teron Village. The village of Ram Teron is five kilometers away from the main Diphu Town. Though the village is situated near to Diphu town, it is lacking behind in infrastructure and development. The village consists of 72 families with a total population of 324 out of which 156 were male and 168 were female. The sex ratio of the female is higher in the village with a sex ratio of 1076 per thousand male. The economy of the majority of the families was totally dependent on natural resources and *jhum* cultivation. The nearest health centre is five kilometers away from the village i.e. the Diphu Civil Hospital but there are medical stores about one kilometer away from the village.

Materials and Method

Among 72 families of Ram Teron village, most of the members were associated with the utilisation of natural herbs and plants to treat their various diseases and health-related problems. The knowledge of Karbi language enabled the author to have an intimate interaction with the studied people. The fieldwork was started from 10th November 2012 and continued up to 15th March 2013. Quantitative data were collected from each household, such as total population, age-sex ratio, economy, literacy etc. Apart from this a few question were ask for each household related with their daily consumption of wild vegetables and about their healthcare practices. Case-studies were taken on the traditional medicine men and the concerned family member associated with the health and diseases.

It focused on their various methods of treatment and also to document some herbs and medicinal plants utilised by the traditional healer to treat various diseases, wounds, and illness. The open structured interview was taken from the eldest person of the village, learned person and the leader of the traditional political organisation. It primarily focused on their concept of health and the role of natural resources in their daily livelihood and culture, moreover on their health, diseases, and treatment. Further, it was also focused on the issue of modern medicine and its impact on the traditional mode of treatment. Participant observation was done by participating in the events of treatment. It has helped the author to know more about their healthcare practices and their ways of treatment, also document some medicinal plants used by the healer. The analysis of data was primarily based on qualitative data, while quantitative data was also used in some cases whenever necessary.

The Karbis Concept of Health and Diseases

Health is the level of functional or metabolic efficiency of a living being. In humans, it is the general conditions of a person's mind and body, usually meaning to be free from illness, injury or pain (as in "good health" or "healthy"). The World Health Organisation (WHO) defined health in its broader sense in 1946 as "a state of complete physical, mental, and social well-being and not merely the absence of disease or infirmity".

The concept of health in Karbi is called *"Ok-pran"* (meaning a state of well-being or unwell). If someone stated that *"Ne-ok-pran mesen"* then he/she is a well or free from illness and if someone stated that *"Ne-ok-pran heno"* then he/she is not well. The Karbis believe that the person who is able to resist illness and able to work for long hours in the field is a healthy person. An obese person is also considered as healthy by some Karbis. Others categorised health as being free from bodily disorder and deformity. However, occasional headache, body pains, minor injury etc. is not considered seriously by the Karbis. In other words, if a person is sufferings from such ailments, he/she would be counted as healthy.

Regarding the concept of diseases, the term *Keso* (illness) is used. The etiology of such *Keso* is supposed to be caused by either natural or by the supernatural forces like the evil eye, the influence of evil spirits, the wrath of gods or deities, breach of taboo, black magic etc. According to their belief, the causation of diseases either natural or supernatural is identified by *Sang-Kelang* (divination) and the person related with the divination is called *Sang-kelang-abang*. Any kind of severe diseases like shivering, severe headache, mental illness etc are supposed to be caused by supernatural forces and the first and foremost is to restore it by rituals. However, diseases like fever, cough, skin diseases, minor injury, cuts wounds, stomach pains, swelling etc. are supposed to be of natural causation and methods of treatment is done either by *Kapherem* (charms) or by applying or consuming some herbs and medicinal plants. Some of the common *charms* practices by the Karbis are *Tharmit Kapherem, Kaipho Kapherem, Ingki Kapherem, Hanso Kapherem, Ok-Kapherem* etc. During the healing process of certain diseases like insect bites, dog bites, wounds cuts by *Kaipho* (*Dendrocalamus hamiltonii*), swelling etc. the performer of the charms (*pherem-bang*) utter some words by narrating the story related with the cause of disease.

Use of Wild Vegetables and Medicinal Plants

The Karbis consumed a number of wild vegetables in their daily dietary habits. These wild vegetables are used either raw or cooked and help to fulfill their daily calories intake. Most of the wild vegetables consumed by the Karbis have a high medicinal value. In the present study, 28 species of wild vegetables and 27 species of medicinal plants use by the Karbis have been recorded. Table 5.1 shows the wild vegetables use by the Karbis with its local and botanical name, also their method of use. Table 5.2 shows the name of the medicinal plant (either single or in combination) use by the Karbis with its local and scientific name, the name of ailment, and methods of preparation and dosages.

Table 5.1: Name of wild vegetables used by the Karbis

Local name	***Scientific Name/Common Name***	***Mode of use***
Han-voti	*Sauropus androgynous Merrill.*	Fried without oil with salt and sesame
Hanmoiso	*Vernonia volkemaefalia*	Leaves cooked with alkaline
Dungkek	*Fern/ Diplazium esculentum*	Leaves boiled in water with salts and sesame
Hanthu	*Gnetum gnemon L.*	Leaves cooled with alkaline
Dido	*Amaranthus viridis*	Fried without oil or with oil
Han-bipo	*Pogostemon parviflorus*	Cooked with alkaline or wrap in a banana leaf and covered with burning charcoal
Tara	*Alpina allughas Retz.*	Cooked with dal, eaten as chutney and boiled in water
Mensopi	*Carica papaya*	Cooked with alkaline, boiled or fried with dal

(Cont'd...)

Ok-hi-atehang	*Homalomena aromatic*	Cooked with alkaline, or cooked with bamboo tubes
Pherklum	*Clerodendrum Colebrook Ian um*	Leaves cooked with salt, dry fish, tomato, and sesame.
Mu-plakplak	*Auricularia auricula-judae*	Cooked with alkaline
Jok-an	*P. thrysiflorus*	Flower boiled with water and eat as chutney
Riho	*Gymnopetalum eochinchinense Kurz.*	Fruit boiled with water are eaten directly or eaten as chutney
Kangkoroi	*Momordica charantia*	Fruits and leaves are eaten as fried or boiled
Rui pharkong		Tuber is boiled or shoved into hot charcoal
Rui-Loru		Tuber is boiled
Hen Salku	*Amorphophallus bulbiferous (Schott) Blume*	Tuber cooked with alkaline or meat etc.
Henru	*Aroids*	Leaves and stem are cooked with water with salt, dry fish, pork, sesame etc.
Mehek	*Rhynchotechum ellipticum*	Cooked with alkaline
Tihaso	*Curcuma aromatic*	Tuber ate as *chutney*
Hanserong	*Hibiscus cannabinus Linn*	Leaves and fruits are cooked with dry fish, meat, sesame etc.
Phi-kangnek	*Alpina galangal (Linn.) Wild*	Leaves Cooked with alkaline and dry fish
Ingsum	*Antidesma acidum Retz.*	Leaves Cooked with salt and dry fish, pork etc.
Tharmit Tharve	*Curcuma amada Roxb.*	Rhizome used as spice or eaten as *chutney*
Hanthai	*Deeringia amaranthoides (Lam.) Merr.*	Fresh rhizome is crush and made into *chutney*
Hanboka	*Olax acuminate Wall. ex Benth*	Tender shoots are eaten boiled
Delap	*Persicaria microcephala (D.Don) H. Gross*	Leaves eaten boiled
Nopak ban	*Oroxylum Indicum (Linn.)*	Leaves eaten boiled

Table 5.2: Name of the medicinal plants used by the Karbis

Local name (single or in combination)	***Scientific name/ Common Name***	***Name of ailment***	***Method of preparation and dosage***
Pherklum	*Clerodendron Colebrookianum Walp.*	High Blood pressure	The fresh leaves are boiled in water and then eaten as vegetables.

(*Cont'd...*)

Tharmit Tharve	*Curcuma amada*	Gastritis	Fresh rhizome juice is taken for remedy
Jok-anso, Noklang (Sugarcane and siluka	*Rauvolfia Serpentina Linn., Terminalia chebulla retz., Sugarcane*	Jaundice	These are mixed with one another and made into pills which are taken thrice daily for five to six days
Delap	*Persicaria microceplala,*	Wounds	Paste of leaves is applied on the affected parts
Kaipho	*Dendrocalamus Hamiltonii*	Cut wounds	Bark is powdered and then applied on the cut wounds to stop bleeding
Rikang menthu	*Paederia foetida Linn.*	Jaundice, dysentery, urinal problem, stomach ache.	Raw leaves juice is taken as a remedy for jaundice, urinal problem and cooked leaves are taken to stop dysentery and stomach ache
Ai-upo	*Costus specious J. Keoning*	Diabetes	Raw leave juice is taken as remedy for Diabetes
Bap Keso	*Amphineurom Opulentum*	Joint pains, backache	Two to three leaves are taken together and then beaten on the pain area
Ingthum abap	*Calotropis gigantia (Linn.) R.Br.ex Ait*	Swelling	Latex is applied on the affected area
Hen Salku	*Amorphophallus bulbiferous (Roxb.) Bl.*	Wounds, allergy affected by Caterpillar	Juice of raw and fresh stem is applied on the affected area
Chipru Abap	*Cassia alata Linn*	Ringworm	Paste leaves are applied on the affected area
Phlek ik and Benvoi	*Clerodendron infortunatum Linn. Gaerti (scientific name not found for Bengvoi)*	Breathing	Leaves of bengvoi and Phlek-ik are boiled and taken as soup
Okhi-atehang	*Homalomena aromatica (Roxb.) Schott*	Joint pain	Paste is applied to the affected part
Chong-amok	*Hydrocotyle sibthorpioides Lam.*	Dysentery	Juice of leaves is taken with meal
Nopak–ban	*Oroxylum indicum (Linn.) Benth*	Intestinal worm	Boiled flowers are taken
Phi-langdung	*Zingiber Zerumbet*	Blood dysentery	Rhizome juice is taken
Siluka	*Terminalia chebulla retz.*	Dysentery, intestinal worm	Fresh or dry fruits are taken
Han-bipo	*Pogostemon Parviflorus*	Joint pains	The leaves are heated on the fire and then applied directly to the joints.

(*Cont'd...*)

Thengsakso	*Murraya Keonigii sprengel*	Gastritis	Leaves juice are taken once daily after meal
Theso Kethor	*Citrus Paradisi Macp.*	Kidney Stone	Fruits juice are mixed with *sobai* (Courie) and then drink
Thebong-kang	*Physalis peruviana Linn.*	Stomach pain	Boiled tender shoots are taken with meal
Han-moiso	*Vernonia Volkemaefalia DC Vern.*	Backache	Leaves are cooked and then eaten with meal
Han-kumphi	*Houttuynia cordata*	Gastritis	Small amount of boiled Leaves is taken with meal
Plim-plam	*Dillenia Indica Linn.*	Hair conditioner	Fruits are applied as hair conditioners
Pharche	*Jatropha*	Toothache	Stems are applied as tooth brush
Pranpri	*Garcinia pedunculata*	Stomach ache, dysentery	Fruits are dried and then mixed with water to drink
Lank-abap	*Acorus Calamus Linn.*	Gastritis	Tuber is eaten as well as tied on the waist

Wild vegetables are mostly collected by the rural women folk. They mostly collected from the forest while going to the field or sometimes they purposely go in search of vegetables. The knowledge of consumption is passing from one generation to another generation and till today they are adopting the same method of consumption. They strongly believe that consuming green leaves gives good digestion and keep them sound health. Today wild vegetables are also available in the local market area.

It was also observed that apart from the traditional healthcare practices the people were also dependent on modern medicine. In the case of severe illness, they go for parallel treatment both from traditional healers and modern healthcare centre.

Belief associated with plants

There are some food taboos observed by the Karbis, among these, the eating of *langdung* (banana flower) and white gourd (*Benincasa hispida*) is strictly forbidden by the Karbi priest. The eating of *Hanjor* and *Chitu* is strictly avoided by the Karbis having *Hem-angtar* (Household deities) and such violation invites divine punishment. The wild plant called *Ingsum* and *Hangjang Chikli* is a taboo for *Engti* and *Terang clan* respectively. It is believed that the plants have once saved their lives during the course of the flood.

Conclusion

Forest and environment is an integral part of tribal life. The tribal utilise the forest resources in multifarious ways i.e. for vegetables, fruits, roots, tubers, medicines etc. Wild plants have been used by the tribal people for ages either for vegetables or for their medicinal purposes. The Karbis are mainly dependent on the natural resources for their daily livelihood. They collect a number of wild plants either from forest or homestead plantation for the preparation of their various cuisine and also for the treatment of their various ailment. But in the present context environmental degradation has put a challenge on their ethnomedicinal practices. It has been found that some of the medicinal plants use by the people has become scarce. Disappearance on the knowledge of medicinal plants could be noticed as the species get exploited. Therefore species that are in traditional herbal practices should be protected because rural communities depend on them. There is an urgent need to study and document their knowledge of future generation. In this regard, more studies on Traditional medicine must be taken in order to impart the knowledge of medicinal plants and to conserve it.

References

Bannerman, RH.1982. 'Traditional medicine in modern healthcare'. *World Forum* 3:8-13.

Baruah, P and GC Sharma.1984. 'Studies on the medicinal uses of plants by the Boro tribal's of Assam'. *J Econ Tax Bot*, 5, 3: 599-604.

Bora, U; A Sahu; AP Saikia; VK Ryakala and P Goswami. 2007. 'Medicinal plants used by the people of Northeast India for curing Malaria'. *Phytotherapy Research,* 21,8:800-804.

Choi, S; M Soopark; YR Lee; TW Kim; SG Do; DS Kim and BH Jean, 2013. 'A standardised bamboo leaf extract inhibits monocyte adhesion to endothelial cells by modulating vascular cell adhesion protein'. *Nature Res Pract* 7, 1: 9-14.

Das, FA; I Barua and DD Das. 2008. 'Ethnomedicinal practices: A case study among the Sonowal Kacharis of Dibrugarh, Assam'. *Ethno-Medicine*, 2, 1:33-37.

Foster, GM and BG Anderson.1978. *Medical Anthropology.* New York Chichester Brisbane, Toronto; John Wiley and Sons.

Gupta, R and KL Chadha 1995. 'Medical and aromatic plants in India'. In KL Chadha and R Gupta (Eds): *Advances in Horticulture: Medical and Aromatic Plants*. pp. 1-44. New Delhi.

Jeetendra, S and AD Kumar 2012. 'Ethnomedicinal plants used by tribal communities for the treatment of snakebite in West Nimar, M. P., India'. *ISCA Journal of Biological Science* 1, 2:77-79.

Krippner, S 2003. 'Models of ethnomedicinal healing'. *Paper Presented at the Ethnomedicine Conferences, Munich, Germany*. April 26–27 and October 11-12.

Lokho, A. 2012. 'The folk medicinal plants of the Mao Naga in Manipur, Northeast India'. *International Journal of Science and Research* 2: 2250-3153.

Lowe, H; A Payne-Jackson; SM Beckstrom-Sternberg and JA Duke. 2000. *Jamaica's Ethnomedicine: Its Potential in the Healthcare System.* pp. 170, University of the West Indies, Kingston, Jamaica; Canoe Press.

Meena, KL and BL Yadav. 2010. 'Studies on ethnomedicinal plants conserved by Garasi tribes of Sirohi district, Rajasthan, India'. *Indian Journal of Natural Products and Resources* 1, 4:500-506.

Srinivasa, BM. 2010. 'Ethnomedical practices among the Jenu Kuruba of Karnataka'. *Man and Life*. 36:107-112.

Tiwari, KC; R Mazumder and S Bhattacharjee.1979. 'Folklore medicines from Assam and Arunachal Pradesh (District Tirap)'. *Quart J Crude Drug Res*, 17, 2:61-67.

World Health Organisation. 2003. *Traditional Medicine*, Fact Sheet No. 134.

Chapter - 6

Natural Resources and Indigenous Knowledge of Healthcare System among the Karbis of Assam

—Somenath Bhattacharjee

Indigenous Knowledge of Healthcare System

Every culture, irrespective of its simplicity and complexity, has its own beliefs and practices concerning diseases. No culture works in a meaningless fashion in its treatment of diseases. Every culture evolves its own system of medicine in order to treat diseases in its own way. This treatment of disease varies from group to group. It has been noted that, in the rural areas, the belief in the interference of a supernatural agency is particularly strong in the context of health and disease. Most of their socio-cultural activities revolve around Gods and Spirits. They identify the supernatural powers with a group of powerful forces and deities which control and influence the happenings in the community. It may be pointed out that disease and treatment, particularly in the simple societies cannot be properly understood in isolation. Health and treatment are very much connected with the environment, particularly the forest ecology. The healthcare system and traditional treatment are based on their deep observation and understanding of nature and environment (Chaudhuri, 2003: 17-24).

Health has been defined in a number of ways. Dubos (1968) defined health as, 'a modus Vivendi enabling imperfect men to achieve a rewarding and too painful existence, while they cope with an imperfect world'. World Health Organisation (1948) defined Health as 'a state of complete physical, mental and social well-being and not merely an absence of disease or infirmity' (Park, 2000:12).

The concept of health, disease, and treatment vary according to the culture of different communities and ethnic groups. Moreover, a particular culture is guided by the traditional customs and every member of the culture is ideally expected to conform to it. Health and disease are universal experiences. Along with the process of human evolution, the diseases were also brought and they become social and cultural facts as well as pathological states. In a given set up for a human being, the disease threatens not only the one's state of well-being and that of other people in the group, but it also threatens the integrity of the community as a whole. In every culture, there is a repository of values and belief systems built around important life experiences viz. birth, illness, and death and disease that reduce the strength of the people to hunt or gather food, to agriculture and all other vital occupational and necessary activities. In such circumstances, the traditional healers had to find a means to prevent misery. The traditional way of treatment is inevitable among the simple societies, although modern treatment is applied in different circumstances. The traditional medicine can be stated as the sum total of all knowledge and practices, whether explicable or not used in diagnosis, prevention and elimination of physical, mental or social imbalance and relying exclusively on practical experiences and observation on. Their traditional medicine is of various kinds like Folk medicine, Ethnomedicine, Ayurveda, Unani, Siddha and Nature Care, which differ from each other in term of tools, techniques, ideas, and beliefs (Banerjee and Jalota, 1988: 18-19).

The anthropological perspective of health is mostly considered under the domain of medical anthropology. It takes up the analysis of health in the context of culture, social behaviour, economic system and human biology. In a sense, medical anthropology is thus a convenient term drawing on a category in our own society, medicine but conceptualised to apply to a broad realm of theory, research and practice that extends well beyond the domain of our own society's licensed medical system. In medical anthropology, the examination of health issues extends to include knowledge, meaning, social behaviour and biology generally related to well-being, suffering misfortune, life cycle and survival (Millard, 1992: 3). It is to be mentioned here that, medical anthropology is not only limited to the extent of providing fruitful strategies to the health planners, but it has its own theoretical dimensions; it is not only a way of viewing the state of health and disease in a society but a way of viewing the society itself. Medical anthropology concerns itself with the many factors that contribute to disease or illness and with the ways that various human populations respond to disease or illness. This perspective views health issues within the context of encompassing political and economic forces that pattern human relationships, shape social behaviour, condition collective experiences, reorder local ecologies and situate cultural meanings including forces of institutional, national and global scale. The roots of medical anthropology are as ancient as the anthropology itself. Medical Anthropology Quarterly, has defined it as a field that includes " ... all inquiries into health, disease, illness, and sickness in human individuals and populations that are undertaken from the holistic and cross-cultural perspective distinctive of anthropology as a discipline- that is with an awareness of species, biological, cultural, linguistic and historical conformity and variation. It encompasses studies of Ethnomedicine, epidemiology, maternal and child health, population, nutrition, human development in relation to health and disease, healthcare providers and services, public health, health policy and the language and speech of health and healthcare" (Medical Anthropology Quarterly: September 2001).

Fabrega 1971, in a definition of medical anthropology, has expressed that a medical anthropology inquiry will be defined as one, " that elucidates the factors, mechanisms, and processes that play a role on or influence the way in which they respond to illness and disease. It also examines these problems with an emphasis on patterns of behaviour."

In most culture, there is a specialist who treats illness, injury, and disease who is also associated with religious practices. Such medico-religious practitioner is also considered to be a practitioner of magic, witchcraft traditionally. Basically, he was a man of cultural mind endowed with many abilities and he was dedicated to his vocation. Throughout the ages, man has been devising ways and means of caring for the sick in the communities. In this context, it is to be mentioned here that, social medicine may be defined as a study of an ill person within his environment with the aim of identifying, classifying and rectifying the causal factors of disease to regain health and later on promote and preserve health. In every culture, there is a substantial and integral body of beliefs, knowledge, and practices built around the major life experiences of health and illness. The constellation of beliefs, knowledge, practices, personal facilities, and resources together from the structure and patterns for the care and treatment of illness of persons of a socio-cultural group is called a medical system. Traditional medicine is defined as "the sum total of all the knowledge and practices, whether explicable or not, used in diagnosis, prevention or elimination of physical, mental or social imbalance and relying exclusively on practical experience and observation handed down from generation to generation whether verbally or in writing. Traditional medicine is not only limited to the arena of treating disease but includes aspects of religion, socio-cultural and economic domains. Traditional societies have always considered the medical practitioners as influential spiritual leaders who handled both the routine and extraordinary medical problems of the society, using magic and religion as the two pivotal rights in their employ, traditional medical practitioners help to conceptualize the ultimate reality of their culture and all the activities they embody (Banerjee and Jalota, 1988: 19). In this context, particularly in India along with the ethnic and cultural diversity, the folk medicine and indigenous knowledge of healthcare system are quite variable from one another.

II

Traditional Healthcare Practices of the Karbi People

The Karbi Anglong District is situated in the central part of Assam. It is bounded by Golaghat district in the east; the State of Meghalaya and Morigaon district in the west; Nagaon and Golaghat district in the north and North Cachar Hill district and the State of Nagaland in the south. The district, with dense tropical forest, covered hills and flat plains were situated between 25^0 33' N to $26^0$35' N Latitude and $92^0$10' to $93^0$50' E Longitude. Due to variation in the topography, this hill zone experiences different climates in different parts. The winter commenced from October and continues till February. During summer, the atmosphere becomes sultry. The temperature ranged from 6 degrees to 12 degrees and 23 degrees to 32 degree Celsius in summer. The average rainfall was about 2416 mm. The population of the district is predominantly tribal. The major tribal groups of this district were Karbis, Bodos, Kukis, Dimasas, Hmars, Garos, Rengma Nagas, Tiwas, and Man etc. Besides, a large number of non-tribals also lived together in this hill region. The Karbis were the indigenous community of the region.

It had the total geographical area of 10,434 sq. kms., which accounts for 13.3 per cent of the total geographical area of the State. It mostly consisted of undulating and hilly terrain with numerous rivers and streams. The district could be broadly divided into two physiographic units, viz. hills and plains. About 85 per cent of the district was covered by the hills. As per the State of Forest Report 1999 of Forest Survey of India, Dehradun, 6044 sq. kms. of the district was under dense forest cover while 2776 sq. km are under open forest cover. The important forest types found in Karbi Anglong District were; moist semi-evergreen forests; moist mixed deciduous forests; riverain type; miscellaneous type with scattered pure or mixed patches of bamboos.

To study the indigenous knowledge of health disease and treatment of the Karbi people, intensive field work was conducted in the selected villages of Karbi Anglong district. The studied areas were one of the oldest settlements of the Karbi people. The study was conducted among 300 families with a total population of 1653. Among them, there were 852 males and 801 females.

The study was conducted during the period of January 2011 to February 2013. Foremostly, the general observation of the village was done along with the completion of preliminary census schedule (PCS) to know the demographic composition of the studied people. Case studies were taken on the concerned families. It was focused on the issues of their historical background, traditional occupational pursuit, present economic pursuit, indigenous knowledge of traditional healthcare practices, magico-religious healing practices. Detailed open structured interviews were taken from the key informant, the eldest person of the settlement, leader of the traditional political organisation of the concerned society, administrative authority related to the studied settlement. It focused on the relevance of locally available floral and faunal resources in their traditional healing practices, a concept about different benevolent and malevolent spirits related to their health aspects. The data were also collected to find out the interaction between cultural and environmental dimensions of healthcare practices among the Karbi people.

The present study is primarily focused on three important aspects, (i) to know about the relationship between man, environment and traditional healthcare practices; (ii) to know about the cultural aspects associated with traditional healthcare practices; and (iii) to know about different local medicinal plants and their importance in the traditional healthcare practices of the concerned people.

Traditional Notion of Illness

The Karbis believe in multiple deities and regards all objects on earth as having divinity or possession of supernatural power and therefore worship hills, mountains, rivers etc. They further believe that diseases are caused by different malevolent spirits and by appeasing the benevolent spirits it can be redressed. Karbis regard both binary spiritual concepts as possessing divinity which can harm as well as bring peace and prosperity to the people such as good health, wealth, favourable weather, etc. Karbis worship household deities called *Hem Angtar* and these deities are propitiated annually. There are deities which are propitiated as and when required are called *Habit ase* (non-household gods).

The disease condition or the notion of illness is being referred by the Karbis as *se kelong*. When a person falls ill, for example, after coming from the forest, the household members attribute the cause due to the encounter of evil spirits and initiates propitiation of the spirits. In case the patient does not respond to normal traditional treatments, the household members seek the help of a wise man to ascertain the cause of the illness. The wise man through divination identifies the deity/spirit responsible for the illness and suggests certain rituals for recovery of the patient. This act of divination is called *sang kelang*. The practice is more prevalent in remote areas where the modern medical facility is a far cry. Sickness, if long continued or severe, is frequently attributed to witchcraft (*Maja*) and the patient is said to be *maja kelong*-witchcraft has got hold of him.

Traditional healthcare practices

Traditional healthcare practices of the Karbis include both local and oral applications and rituals to cure a host of diseases like anemia, muscular inflammation, pain (analgesia), etc. *Keso* or illness is also called *se kelong*, a generic term for contracting illnesses and its treatment is called *se kelang*. *Se kelang* therefore, involves numerous sacred healing incantations, chants, prayers and rituals and in some cases administration of plant and animal products. The rituals may be widely divided into (a) *kapherem* and (b) *karkli*. In *kapherem*, a cure for certain *keso* (pain or illness) is sought by performing healing chants involving the external application of saliva of the mouth (*kehi / kangthok*) and mild blowing of air (*kebut*) on the afflicted portion of the body. *Kapherem* is performed for the cure of numerous pain or *keso* such as (1) *Ingki angmi* (toxins of caterpillars), (2) *Bap ase*, (3) *Ingthum* (boils/furuncle), (4) *Methan kekor* (dog bite), (5) *Pok avur* (epidemic of stomach disease), (6) *But Pharo* (acute stomach ache), (7) *Chor kedong* (thorn inflicted injury), (8) *Me kapherem* (burn), (9) *Inghai* (lymphadenitis), (10) *Han kangri* (vegetable poisoning), (11) *Sor kapherem* (acute pain), (12) *Mek avur* (epidemic of eye disease), (13) *Chainong a-but* (acute stomach pain), (14) *Thengkur* (poisoning) and (16) *Phurui kangthok* (snake bite) etc. to cite a few. In *kapherem*, blood-sacrifice is generally not involved. In extreme cases when the *keso* does not respond to *kapherem*, blood-sacrifice or *karkli* is resorted to. Philosophically, therefore, in traditional Karbi healing system, blood-sacrifice is not the first option.

In *karkli*, a priest resorts to the reading of entrails and liver of sacrificed chickens, goats or pigs. This practice of divining, known since the time of ancient Etruscans, Romans, and the Mesopotamians is known as *haruspicy*, *hepatoscopy* or *hepatomancy*, the inspection of the entrails of sacrificed animals, especially the livers of sacrificed sheep and poultry. The practice is also known as 'extispicy (from Latin extispicium), the practice of using anomalies in animal entrails to predict or divine future events. Organs inspected include the liver, intestines, and lungs. The animal used for extispicy must often be ritually pure and slaughtered in a special ceremony'. Besides the reading of the entrails and livers etc., the direction of the head and wings of the sacrificed chicken is also examined. Karbi people use a number of locally available plant resources to redress their different ailments. The collection of such resources, its purification and further the method related to the preparation of medicine from them, are an integral part of their cultural tradition, customs, and taboo. A few of such plants and their specific utilisation are mentioned below:

Table 6.1: Floral resources utilised by the Karbi as medicinal resources

Botanical name of the plant	*Local name*	*Consumed for*	*Method of use and dosage*
Abrus precatorius Linn.	*Chuselok*	Cough	Two tablespoons of fresh juice, twice daily after meals for six days.
Acmella paniculata	*Bapchuki*	Stomach ache	One tablespoon of leaf juice is taken after meals, twice daily for five days.
Adhatoda zeylanica	*Jok –an-kelok*	Dysentery	Juice of two matured leaves, thrice daily before a meal for three days.
Alpinia galanga	*Phrikangnek*	Bronchitis	Half a teacup of rhizome juice, once daily after meal for ten days.
Alternanthera sessilis	*Raeaba*	Skin disease	Fresh leaves paste applied on the affected parts twice daily for eight days.
Amorphophallus bulbiferous	*Hen saiku*	Piles	100 g tuber boiled and taken with rice twice daily for a month.
Antidesma acidum	*Ingchum*	Appetizers	Two boiled tender shoots were taken with rice, once a day for five days.
Arisaema tortuosum	*Chamua*	Piles	50 g tuber boiled and taken with rice, twice daily for a month.
Beta vulgaris	*Bengali dido*	Jaundice	50 g boiled tender shoots taken once a day with a meal for ten days.
Calamus rotang	*Pri*	Vitality	50 g boiled tender shoots taken with a meal for twenty days.

(*Cont'd...*)

Cassia tora	*Bapduli*	Jaundice	Five tablespoons of leave juice once daily after meal for fifteen days.
Chenopodium album	*Churu*	Dysentery	Two tablespoons of leave juice thrice daily after a meal.
Cissus quandragularis	*Repichingthun*	Joint pain	25gm of boiled stem taken with a meal once daily for ten days.
Clerodendrum serratum	*Phelang-riho*	Wound	Matured fruits are crushed and make into a paste and then applied on the affected parts.
Commelina benghalensis	*Kurveng*	Earache	Two drops of leaf juice are applied on the affected ear once daily for three days.
Curcuma amada	*Tharmit tharve*	Gastritis	Two table spoon full of rhizome juice twice daily after meal for five days.
Cycas pectinata	*Or –oh*	Gastritis	Three tablespoons of leaf juice twice daily after meal for five days.
Drymaria cordata	*Kur-vengso*	Sinusitis	Two drops of warm leaf juice are applied as drops once daily for six days.
Homalomena aromatica	*Ok hi atehang*	Joint pain	Petiole paste applied on the affected parts twice daily for a month.
Lippia geminata	*Lopong brik*	Conjunctivitis	One drop of leaf juice applied once daily for three days.
Nyctanthes arbor-tristis	*Hewali*	Malaria	Half a teacup of leaf juice once daily after meal for ten days.
Oroxylum Indicum	*Nopak ban*	Intestinal worm	Two boiled flowers twice daily after meal for seven days.
Solanum nigrum	*Pharchingki*	Intestinal worm	Three matured fruits once daily after a meal.
Physalis peruviana	*Thebongkang*	Stomach pain	25 g of boiled tender shoot taken with a meal once a day for five days.
Paederia foetida	*Rikang menthu*	Gastritis	Four tablespoons full of leaf juice, once daily after meal for a week.
Vitex negundo	*Vorke abap*	Malaria	50 g leaves boiled in 300 ml water till the quantity become half and then taken twice daily after meals for fifteen days.
Xanthium strumarium	*Parok hanthor*	High blood pressure	225 g of boiled shoot taken with a meal twice daily for twenty days.
Zingiber zerumbet	*Phrilangdung*	Blood dysentery	Two tablespoons of rhizome juice taken after a meal for five days.

Source: Field Study, 2011-2013.

Meanwhile, fish is symbolically used in almost all Karbi rituals and it plays a very crucial role in the traditional healthcare practices of the Karbi people.

Ritualistic use of fish

All rituals are associated with various healing practices or general well-being of individuals, household or village communities which are performed either at home, within the boundary of a village or in the woods (in a safe distance from the village). Fish is symbolically used in all the healing practices. Fish (of any species) is collected from rivers (or from ponds these days) one day ahead of the ritual and brought home which is then cooked (only boiled without adding any flavour or salt). The boiled fish is then wrapped in a leaf and tied with nine strands of *jintak* (fine bamboo stripes). The fish thus sanctified is called *beng* which is offered at the altar where the particular deities are worshipped.

Beng is used in the rituals for *Hem angtar* or household deities such as *Peng*, *Rong Arnam*, *Chojun,* and *Rongker*. In the beginning of the ritual, the *Kurusar* or priest pay compliance and honour to his predecessors by offering rice beer followed by *beng*. By this practice, the *kurusar* is said to inform his *kuru* or predecessors that the former is performing the ritual acquired from them and did not act unilaterally and ask for blessings for smooth conduct of the ritual. Ritual without honouring the *kuru* by the *kurusar* is said to be incomplete. *Beng* or sanctified fish is not offered at rituals generally performed in the woods called *bit-ase* such as *duikrai* or *chekama*.

During *Chojun*, the supreme deity of Karbi pantheon *Arnam kethe* (variously known as *Barithe, Abinong*, *Athak asor* etc.) is offered live fish or *ok-kereng* of two varieties namely *nune* (*Amblypharyngodon mola, Danio aequipinnatus*) and *ok-langso* (*Channa gachua*) along with *chehe* (*Carcinus* sp.) and *kumphi* (*Dytiscus marginalis*).

Use of fish to cure mental depression (*Nihu kachingtung*)

Karbis are organised around a network of kinship relations. The maternal uncles are held in high esteem in Karbi society and traditionally, it is customary for all sisters to pay periodic homage/obeisance to their brothers. When a sister's son/daughter is afflicted with certain socially defined abnormalities, they approach a '*sang kelang abang*' or a diviner who performs certain rituals to identify the particular brother (elder or younger) who is to be ritually propitiated. This ceremony /ritual are called *Nihu kachingtung* or *nihu kachiri* (longing of maternal uncle).

The particular *nihu* (maternal uncle) is approached, offered customary wine, who will then give six fist-full of rice and six pieces of *toman* (dried fish prepared out of bigger varieties of fish of any species) for the afflicted person. The quantity of ritual gift is five fist-full of rice and five pieces of *toman* if the afflicted person is female and six fist-full of rice and six pieces of *toman* if the afflicted person is male. If the person partakes the ritual gifts (of rice and *toman*), the abnormalities are said to be cured.

Fish as Ethnomedicine

Fishes are used to address a host of health-related disorders such as a cough, anemia, etc among different tribes of Karbi Anglong district namely Karbi, Dimasa and Thadou tribes. Some fishes are avoided during certain illnesses, for example, among the Karbis; the patient suffering from throat problem, goiter or leprosy is barred from eating scaled fishes. Tuberculosis patients are barred from eating all fishes. Similarly, among the Dimasas the patient suffering from skin ailments are barred from eating *Pontius* sp., *Walllago atu* is also avoided during illnesses and during urinary tract infection the head of the fish is avoided. The following table will give an in-depth view of the utilisation of locally available fishes by the Karbi people for their numerous ailments were also observed that the villagers

Table 6.2: Utilisation of locally available fishes by the Karbi

Scientific name	*Local name*	*Tribe*	*Parts used*	*Disease condition*	*Application*
Danio aequipinnatus	*Nune*	Karbis	Whole fish	Constant spitting or *ingthokset*	The boiled fish is consumed regularly.
Monopterus cuchia	*Kumchirui*	Karbis	Whole fish or raw blood	Anaemia	Raw blood is taken orally.
		Karbis	Whole fish/blood	Kalazar	Small sized raw fish is taken orally or fresh blood of the fish is consumed.
		Karbis	Blood	Entry of leech	Fresh blood is consumed raw as tonic for removal of leech from rectum/anus.
Puntius sp.	*Ok-puthi*	Karbis	Head	Night-blindness	The cooked head is taken regularly.
Clarius batrachus	*Nagur*	Karbis	Whole fish	Smallpox	Cooked fish is eaten.
Mystus sp.	*Tengera*	Karbis	Whole fish	Smallpox	Cooked fish is eaten.

(*Cont'd...*)

Any hillstream fish		Karbis	Belly	Sore festering wounds	The affected area is bandage with fish belly and kept for 2-3 days.
Channa gachua	*Ok-langso*	Karbis	Bile	When pricked by thorn	The bile of the fish is applied when pricked by a thorn, it becomes easy to remove.
Puntius sp. (fermented)	*Manthu*	Karbis	Whole fish	Blood purifier	*Manthu* is cooked with bamboo shoot and taken.
				Common cold	Manthu is cooked with chili and taken to cure a common cold.
Anguilla bengalensis	*Nujung*	Karbis	Fats	Rheumoid-arthritis	The fats are used as an ointment.
Heteropnue-stes fossils	*Singki*	Karbis	Brain	Sting by the fish itself	The brain of the fish is used as an antidote. The brain is consumed raw when stung by the fish itself.
Wallago atu	*Seketa*	Karbis	Head	To maintain health of the liver	Boiled head of the fish is taken regularly.
Labeo pangusia	*Notun*	Karbis	Flesh of the fish	Weakness after delivery	Boiled fish is taken regularly.
		Karbis	Bile	Stomach ache	Bile of the fish is taken orally.
Channa punctatus	*Ok-meklot/ ok-borok*	Karbis	Eyes	Corn or clavus	The eyes of the fish are mixed with common salt applied to the corn affected part of the body.

had a strong belief related with the influence of soul for different health anomaly. They had a strong faith on the malevolent impact of evil wind, evil eye, and charming arrow. The only way to get rid of the ill health condition is to please the soul with magico-religious performances. Such performances were conducted with sacrifices of animals, with a strong faith that it will redress the evil effect of the soul on different ill health condition. The sacrifices were usually performed by the magico-religious healers of the village.

The Karbis regard both Gods and Devils as possessing divinity which can do harm as well as bring peace and prosperity to the people. In this concern, a number cultural norm is associated with their reproductive mother-child health issues. A prospective mother is supposed to walk across the river, streams, and hilly areas, with the belief that through such movements she will be blessed by nature. It is a cultural taboo for her to consume the flesh of tortoise or chameleon. They believe that complicated situations during pregnancy occur due to the curse of an evil spirit known as *Hi-i-phuri.* In such cases, a wise man sacrifices a cock and offers the blood to the evil spirit. Just before one month of the expected delivery, the concerned families invite a wise man to perform the *Voti-langpon kevar* ritual to prevent the influence of any evil spirit that may cause hindrance during pregnancy. Ultimately it is obvious that a number of cultural practices and environmental resources are intimately related to the traditional healthcare practices of the Karbi people.

Table 6.3: Influence of malevolent soul causing ailment

Name of the Soul or Spirit	***Category (M/F)***	***Cause of Disease***	***Redressal Method***
Karjong (Soul) of a human being.	Both male and female	The Karbi concept on soul was found to be known as *Karjong* and it is believed that in term of mental disorder, Peculiarity behaviour is the cause of disease which occurred when a person soul is a trap by the evil spirit. It is done for bringing harm to the person.	The *Kurusar* (religious practitioner) find the cause and the *Sekarkli* (ritual is performed) like sacrificing of animals.
Chamburukso is a spirit which exists after a person's death.	Both male and female	*Chamburukso* prevails after a person dies. This spirit tries to disturb any one of his friend/ relatives when he is unsatisfied for anything at the time of his death. Through certain sign at the time of any ritual ceremony that takes place at home, Tries to harm or disturbed his relative with certain sign a person feel discomfort, uneasiness occurred, sometimes a person feels cold and faint.	In order to avoid such situation, a small piece of banana leaves as plates are placed on the ground for as many *Chamburukso* or ancestor spirit and wine sprinkled and pieces of burnt dried fish offered by an elder member who chants incantation praying for their blessing.

The fundamental universal concept of healthcare practices is to cure and prevent diseases and illness. Ever since the attainment of culture building capacity by man, there have been attempts to devise cures for multifarious diseases. Man since his emergence remained engaged in attempting to combat different fatal diseases. Folk medicine has served this purpose over the last 3,000 years or so in India. In the historic past at all levels of socio-cultural development, there could hardly be any group of the population that has not had its own concept of health, disease, and treatment. The people of a habitation region, in general, become knowledgeable about the curative or preventive medicinal plant species abounding in the region. The concerned people are apt to learn the utility of some herbs available near at hand. The people living in the sub-mountainous region of Karbi Anglong, as sedentary inhabitants, came into intimate contact with various geophysical features and the environment. Simultaneously, they gain a distinctive knowledge of the total environs of the habitat. The Karbi people used a large number of medicinal plants for their self-therapy. Besides the use of different herbs by common people, the traditional healers had the knowledge to use the herbal medicine and to diagnose the bodily disorders. Such traditional healing practices are acclaimed to have classic effective value on account of their being non-toxic, non-cost worthy and easy availability. Further, a number of physical ailments were attributed to different supernatural causes. Different magico-religious practices were widely conducted to cure such maladies.

The concerned people had a strong faith on evil eye, evil wind, and charming arrow. To redress the malevolent effect of such evil forces a number of magico-religious healing practices were performed by the magico-religious practitioners of the studied area. Even the elderly members of the concerned community also had the knowledge about different magico-religious healing practices. It is to be mentioned here that economic scarcity was a major hindrance for the studied people to avail the modern medical treatment. In such circumstance the environmental resources and cultural practices had played a major role in their traditional healthcare system; as well as an intimate psychological dependency could be also noticed on it.

References

Banerjee, BG and R Jalota, 1988. *Folk Illness and Ethnomedicine,* New Delhi; Northern Book Centre.

Chaudhuri, B. 2003. *Health, Forest, and Development: The Tribal Situation*. New Delhi; Inter-India Publication.

Dubos, R. 1968. *Man, Medicine and Environment*. Harmondsworth; Pelican.

Fabrega, H. 1971. 'Medical Anthropology'. In BJ Siegal (Ed): *Biennial Review of Anthropology*. pp.1-2. Stanford; Stanford University Press.

Millard, AV. 1992. 'The anthropological analysis of health'. *Medical Anthropology Quarterly* 6, 1: 3-5.

Ministry of Environment and Forest. 1999. *Forest Survey of India*. Dehradun; Government of India.

Park, K 2000. *Park's Textbook of Preventive and Social Medicine* (21st edition), Jabalpur; Banarasidas Bhanot Publishers.

Chapter - 7

Ethno-medicine among the Sonowal Kachari of Assam

—Dali Dutta and Sarthak Sengupta

Introduction

Ethnomedicine is a sub-field of medical anthropology and deals with the study of traditional medicines; not only those that have relevant written sources (e.g. traditional Chinese medicine, Ayurveda) but especially those, whose knowledge and practices have been orally transmitted over the centuries. Ethnomedicine refers to 'those beliefs and practices relating to disease which are the products of indigenous cultural development and is not explicitly derived from the conceptual framework of modern medicine' (Hughes, 1968). In recent times with the increased knowledge of life and culture of the indigenous communities, the social scientists are taking interest in ethnomedicinal studies.

The ethnomedicinal systems have two universal categories of disease: a natural illness that explains illness in impersonal systemic terms. Thus, the disease is thought to stem from natural forces or conditions such as cold, heat and possibly by an imbalance in the basic body elements. Unnatural illnesses are caused by two major types of supernatural forces. One is caused due to the result of evil spirits or human agents using sorcery and spiritual causes that are the results of sins, breaking taboos or caused by God.

In India, few works in this regard (Choudhury, 1986; Bhadra and Tirkey, 1997 and many others) have been reported ethnomedical practices especially from among the rural and tribal communities of India. Ray and Sharma (2005) have given a vivid description of ethnomedicinal beliefs and practices prevalent among the Savaras, a tribal community of Andhra Pradesh.

Significant contribution towards the understanding of some isolated population of North East India in this regard was attempted by Saikia (1964), Pulu (1979), Dutta Choudhury and Ghosh (1984), Bhowmik and Pal (1984), Barua (1984), and Guha (1986) has reported from among the Dafla, Idu Mishmi, Nocte, Kaman Mishmi and Boro-Kachari tribe of North East India respectively. A glimpse of indigenous health practices among the plain tribes of Assam is given by Sharma Thakur (1999). The studies by Jain and Borthakur (1980), Medhi (1995), Dutta and Nath (1999), Medhi and Paul (2004), Bhardwaj and Gakhar (2005), Das and Tag (2006), Sajem and Gosai (2006), Buragohain and Konwar (2007), Das *et al.*, (2008), Kalita and Bora (2008), and Saikia *et al.*, (2010) are to name a few.

The socio-economic condition and the problems related to health and indigenous methods of treatment of some of the tribes of Arunachal Pradesh has been reported by Choudhury (2000), Duarah and Pathak (1997), Kohli (1999), Bhasin (1997, 1999, 2002, 2003 and 2005).

The Sonowal Kachari is a plains Scheduled Tribe of Assam. They mainly inhabits in Dibrugarh, Lakhimpur, Dhemaji, Tinsukia, Jorhat and Golaghat districts of Upper Assam. According to 2001 census, the Sonowal Kachari population is 2, 35,881 which is roughly 7.10 per cent of the total scheduled tribe population in the State of Assam. They belong to the Tibeto-Burman linguistic family but at present, they had adopted the Assamese language. Agriculture is the main occupation of the Sonowal Kacharis. They are mostly cultivators.

Material and Methods

In this study, an attempt has been made to find out the beliefs and practices related to healthcare system among the population under study. Data for the present study were collected from Chelajan Kachari village of Lakhimpur district of upper Assam. The information collected covers two major aspects of indigenous health practices viz., (i) preventive healthcare including cleanliness, sanitation and hygiene, nutrition and food habits, family planning, and midwifery, death, and disposal of dead bodies and (ii) ethnomedicine including traditional concepts, spiritual beliefs and practices relating to diseases and therapy. Some of the information under the first category was collected by observation. Information on the diseases and their respective curves were collected from the knowledgeable persons and village medicine men, who are regularly consulted by the villagers. Information thus collected were checked and verified from the persons who had suffered earlier or have been suffering at the time of inquiry.

Diseases and treatments

The Sonowal Kachari possesses very rich traditional knowledge of indigenous medicine. They have their own methods of treating different kinds of diseases, using locally available herbs and plants for treatment; following the knowledge inherited from their ancestors. The medicine men are referred by a different term. They are popularly called as *Bez* and in rural Assam, they are mainly known by this term. They are ordinary cultivators but have a respectable position in the society. They do not demand any remuneration, but usually, they are offered honorarium consists of *pan tambul* (betel nut and vine) and token money. It has been observed that the use of herbal medicine for curing certain diseases are quite known to the people and besides medicine-men, many elderly persons also know about the use of herbal medicines. The ethnomedicine practitioners treat the individual holistically and consult the root cause of their illness. Different herbal remedies are prescribed for each patient's specific needs.

The data included the types of diseases with its local name, besides curatives of vegetative and animal origin. Some of the diseases and their indigenous methods of treatments are as follows:

1. *Nose bleed:* To bring immediate relief from this ailment, the flower of pomegranate (*Punica granatum Linn*), crushed and 3-4 drops of juice are poured into the nose.
2. *Tonsillitis:* By mixing seed of *Amara (Sponolias mangifera)*, a seed *Silikha (Terminalia chebula*) and a piece of turmeric (*Curcuma domestica*) a juice is prepared and counseling the patient to gargle for a week regularly.
3. *Pain in the ear:* To cure ear-ache, juice of *Tulsi (Ocimum sanctum),* boiled and placed in the ear.
4. *Fever:* To get relief from fever, lime (*Citrus aurantifolia*) juice is mixed with sugar and applied on the forehead of the patient.
5. *Diarrhoea:* To cure the disease, bark of long pepper mixed with *misiri* water is used. Another medicine is also used by the Sonowal Kachari that is dry gooseberry (*Embica officinalis gaertin*) powder and black salt mixed with cold water is taken.
6. *Dysentery:* To cure this disease, the juice of black *Tulsi* leaves (*Ocimum sanctum*) and *Sirata* (*Swertia chirata*) is used. Lime (*Citrus aurantifolia*) juice with hot water and a little salt is also used in dysentery. For the blood dysentery the juice of tender leaves (three numbers) of mango (*Mangifera indica*), blackberry (*Suzycium cuminii L.*) and gooseberry (*Emblica officinalis gaeetin*)

in equal proportions together with honey is mixed with goat milk is taken. Honey together with the juice of *Dubari* grass (*Cynodon dactylon*) can cure blood dysentery. It needs to be taken consecutively for three/four days. The juice of *Manimuni* (*Centella asiatica*), mixed with sugar or honey should be taken continuously for a month to cure the disease. They also use lime-water (*chun pani*) mixed with the juice of turmeric leaf (*Curcuma domestica*) to get relief from blood dysentery and mucous.

7. *Jaundice:* The medicine is prepared by pounding five or six number of *Silikha* (*Terminalia chebula*) mixing with jaggery and they believe it can cure jaundice. A glass of sugarcane (*Saccharum officinarum*) juice twice daily prescribed for the purpose. Boiled raw papaya (*Carica papaya*) is said to be good for curing the disease. *Kordoi* (*Averrhoa carambola*), Goose Berry (*Emblica officinalis gaertin*), Sugar cane (*Saccharun officinarum*), *Neem* leaves (*Azadirachta indica*), *Duran ban* (*Leucas cephalotes spreng*), *Brahmi sak* (*Bacopa monnieri*), *Purakol* (*Musa paradisiaca*) are prescribed edibles for the patient.
8. *Blood Vomiting:* Blood vomiting can be cured with a tablespoon of carrot juice (*Daucus carota*) mixed with honey.
9. *Liver Disease:* A curry prepared from the inflorescence of banana (*Musa paradisiaca*) and the meat of pigeon is used as a medicine to cure liver disease. Two to three pieces of papayas (*Carica papaya*) also consumed daily for the purpose.
10. *Worms:* To get relief from worms, the twigs of *Chirata* (*Swertia chirata*) are soaked in the water overnight and the water is prescribed to drink in empty stomach in the morning for one week regularly. A paste of five lemon seeds mixed with water is also prescribed to eat in empty stomach for a few days.
11. *Scabies:* To remove scabies, the Sonowal Kachari people take bath with hot water in which leaves of *Neem* (*Azadirachta officinarum*) were boiled. Lemon juice mixed with coconut oil is massaged for curing scabies. Twigs of *Chirata* (*Swertia chirata*) are crushed into a paste with water to be used as an ointment and applied on the skin. *Chirata* water is prescribed to drink in the morning in empty stomach.
12. *Piles:* An Edible portion of a ripe mango (*Mangifera indica*) with a small amount of rhizomatous stem of ginger is given to take twice daily for a week. After removing the outer portion of modified root of radish (*Raphanus sativus*) is allowed to insert

into the rectum and kept as such for the whole night. Next morning the used portion is removed and the area is cleaned with extract of rhizomatous stem of ginger. It is repeated every week until cured.

13. *Lice control:* The juice extracted from the leaves of *Pategoja* is applied over the scalp for 15 minutes for the treatment. It is repeated at five days intervals for a month. Fruit of *Datura* is also applied for the same treatment.
14. *Diabetes:* The bark of *Chajina* (*Moringa oleifera*) is crushed with a small amount of water and the extracted juice is given thrice daily for a week.
15. *Paralysis:* Young shoots of *Bhedai lata* (*Echites fructes cens*) are crushed and extracted juice is given for message until cure.
16. *Asthma:* The edible portion of the rhizomatous stem of *Naharu (Allium sativum*) is crushed and mixed with a glass of raw milk of cow and given to drink early in the morning for a week.
17. *Glossities:* The juice extracted from young leaves of *Madhuri* (*Psidium guayava*) is applied over the infected tongue twice daily for three days.
18. *Mumps:* Young shoots of *Akon* (*Calotropis gigantea*), *Laijabori* (*Drymaria cordata*) and *Dimoru* (*Ficus glomerata*) are crushed together and extracted juice is used on the infected portion.

The spiritual aspect of health and sickness has been an integral component of the ethnomedicinal practice for centuries. The Sonowal Kachari people also believed that magico-religious beliefs, any breach of taboos, witchcraft are the agents of ill health. Mystical powers like the evil eye, evil mouth and evil touch are also believed to be the agents of diseases.

Magical practices are performed on various occasions to keep the people and society free from the danger of any health hazards. They believe that each spirit has its own myth and it is closely related to various aspects of life. Generally, traditional beliefs, traditional healers, and traditional medicines play a very prominent role in supporting and maintaining health in the rural Sonowal Kachari villages. Some of these are given below:

1. *Aii nam*: It is believed that Goddess Parvati appears in the form of *'aii'* and she bears various epithets like Durga, Mahamaya, Bhagavati, Sitala etc. depending upon her missions on earth. She causes various diseases, fever, headache, stomach pain etc.

To get relief from these diseases the Sonowal women offer prayer towards the '*Aii*' and put forward betel nut and vine and other raw materials.

2. *Akhan pota nam*: When a man/woman is suffering from chicken pox, then the womenfolk of the village visits that house wearing a white dress and offer *tamul pan, salita, payash* and prays to '*Aii.*'
3. *Lakhimi nam*: The main occupation of Sonowal Kachari is agriculture. Therefore, they pray Goddess Lakhimi for the bumper cropping of their paddy.
4. *Aapesara nam*: Witch, evil spirits, fairies live in the pond causes various diseases. So, for the welfare of the people and society, the women of the village sing *aapesara nam* near the river or pond offering betel nut and lighting the earthen lamp.
5. *Ayukh tula sobah*: This *sobah* is observed when one person gets frightened from an accident or for any other reasons, then to get relief the Sonowal Kachari people perform this ceremony. Although this ceremony is observed by women, however one or two male people are allowed to participate. Usually, this is performed either in the dusk or in the early night.
6. *Aapesara sobah*: The Sonowal Kachari people believe that serious conditions arise out of any disease is caused due to the fury of the fairy (*Aapesari*). So when a family member is suffering from eye problem or stomach problem then with the help of at least five women they propitiated the fairy and offered powdered rice, milk, betel nut, vine and token money.
7. *Bator sobah*: For an overall prosperity of the village and to get relief from the diseases, the people perform this *sobah*. This is usually held in the two ends of the village and the required raw materials are powder rice, sugar, betel nut and vine.
8. *Gopini sobah*: For the well-being of the village people more particularly for curing various diseases and to get rid of accidents this *sobah* is held at *Namghar* (prayer house) for three consecutive days. Soaked gram, banana, betel nut, vine and earthen lamp are offered.
9. *Bhur utua sobah*: This is a community level worship. To get relief from the diseases this *sobah* is organised. One pair of betel nut and leaf is offered from each family. One red duck is offered on behalf of the villagers. All the offered articles are placed on a

raft made out of plantain and then the *bhur* is float (*utua*) in the river with the help of four men.

Thus, it is apparent from the study that supernatural or magico-religious cures amongst the Sonowal Kachari invariably involve rituals and prayers for invoking the spirits.

Conclusion

The healthcare practices and system of treating diseases amongst the Sonowals are based on their deep surveillance and belief in nature. However, with the introduction of formal education and their awareness towards the importance of health and healthcare practices and also with the advent of modern healthcare facilities which includes different health measures and facilities offered by the government, nowadays, the Sonowals are becoming more interested in taking modern medicine instead of traditional herbal medicine. Among the Sonowal Kachari, the knowledge of traditional medicine, which they preserve for centuries, is dying with the elders. Therefore, textualisation of this dying wisdom and scientific assessment of its relevance in the contemporary situation is urgently needed. It is observed that the upcoming generations are fast becoming dependent on modern medicine. As a result, interesting intermixing of a different system of healthcare practices in recent days leads to medical pluralism and calls for urgent attention. Time has come to take immediate step to protect the Intellectual Property Rights (if any) of the people under study. An inter-disciplinary effort to find out various problems and prospects associated with this field of research is also expected.

References

Barua S. 1984. 'A study of indigenous health practices among the Kaman Mishmis of Lohit district of Arunachal Pradesh'. *Human Science*, 33, 4: 232-244.

Bhadra RK and JB Tirkey. 1997. 'Health culture practices in rural society: Case studies of castes and tribes of North Bengal', In F. Ahmed Das and RK Kar (Eds.): *Health Studies in Anthropology*. pp 79-94; Dibrugarh University, Dibrugarh; Department of Anthropology, Dibrugarh University, Assam.

Bhardwaj S and SK Gakhar. 2005. 'Ethnomedicinal plants used by the tribals of Mizoram to cure cuts and wounds'. *Indian Journal of Traditional Knowledge*, 4, 1: 75.

Bhasin V. 2005. 'Tribals of Ladakh: Ecology and health'. *Stud. Tribes Tribals,* 3: 1-13.

Bhasin V. 1997. 'Medical pluralism and health services in Ladakh'. *J. Soc. Sci.,* 1: 43-69.

Bhasin, V. 1999. *Tribals of Ladakh: Ecology, Human Settlements, and Health*. Delhi; Kamala-Raj Enterprises.

Bhasin, V. 2002. 'Traditional medicine among tribals of Rajasthan'. *J. Soc Sci.,* 6, 3: 153-172.

Bhasin, V. 2003. 'Sickness and therapy among tribals of Rajasthan'. *Stud. Tribes and Tribals*, 1, 1: 77 -83.

Bhowmik, DC and A Pal, 1984, 'Indigenous health practices among the Noctes of Arunachal Pradesh', *Human Science*, 33, 1: 35-53.

Buragohain, J and BK Konwar, 2007. 'Ethnomedicinal plants used in skin diseases by some Indo-Mongoloid communities of Assam'. *Asian J Exp Sci*, 21, 2: 281-288.

Choudhury, B. 1986. 'Medical Anthropology in India with special reference to tribal populations', In B Choudhury (Ed): *Tribal Health: Socio-Cultural Dimensions*, New Delhi; Inter-India Publications.

Choudhury, S. 2000. 'Indigenous beliefs and practices of herbal medicine among the few Arunachal'. *Resarun*, 26: 72-81.

Das, AK and H Tag. 2006. 'Ethnomedicinal studies of the Khamti tribe of Arunachal Pradesh'. *Indian Journal of Traditional Knowledge*, 5, 3: 317-322.

Das, FA, I Barua and DD Das, 2008. 'Ethnomedicinal practices: A case study among the Sonowal Kacharis of Dibrugarh, Assam'. *Ethno-Med*, 2, 1: 33-37.

Duarah, DK and SD Pathak. 1997. 'A short note on the healthcare practices among the Nishis of Arunachal Pradesh', In F Ahmed Das and RK Kar (Eds.): *Health Studies in Anthropology*. pp. 73-78. Department of Anthropology, Dibrugarh University, Dibrugarh.

Dutta Choudhury, SS and GC Ghosh, 1984, 'Indigenous health practices among the Idu Mishmis of Arunachal Pradesh'. *Human Science*, 33, 1: 24-34.

Dutta, M and SC Nath. 1999. 'Ethno-medico botany of the Tai-Ahoms of Assam, India'. *Journal of Econ Taxon Bot,* 23, 2: 591-598.

Guha, A. 1986. 'Folk medicines of the Boro-Kacharis – A plain tribe of Assam', In B. Chaudhuri (Ed.): *Tribal Health*. pp 191-199. New Delhi; Inter-India Publications.

Hughes, Charles C 1968. 'Ethnomedicine', In *International Encyclopedia of the Social Sciences.* Vol.X. London: Crowell Collier and Macmillan Inc.

Jain, SK and SK Borthakur 1980. 'Ethnobotany of Mikirs of India'. *J Econ Taxon Bot*, 34: 264-272.

Kalita, D. and RL Bora. 2008. 'Some folk medicines from Lakhimpur district, Assam'. *Indian Journal of Traditional Knowledge*, 7, 3: 414-416.

Kohli, YP. 1999. 'Herbal medicines in Arunachal Pradesh', In S Sengupta (Ed.), *Health, Healers, and Healing: Studies in Medical Anthropology*. pp. 258-264. Dibrugarh: N. L. Publications.

Medhi, BK 1995. 'Ethnomedicine: A study among the Mishings in a rural context'. *Bulletin of the Department of Anthropology,* Guwahati University, 9: 61-68.

Medhi, BK and B Paul. 2004. 'Health and hygiene of the Nahs of Arunachal Pradesh'. *Stud Tribes Tribals*, 2, 1: 23-27.

Pulu, J. 1979, 'The plants those are used by the Idus of Lohit district for medicinal purposes'. *Resarun,* 5, 2: 10-14.

Ray, A and BV Sharma, 2005. 'Ethnomedical beliefs and practices among the Savara', In S. Sahay and PK Singh (Eds.): *Dimensions of Researches in Indian Anthropology*. Vol. II, pp. 454-464, New Delhi; Serial Publications.

Saikia, B; SK. Borthakur and N. Saikia 2010. 'Medico-ethnobotany of Bodo tribals in Gohpur of Sonitpur district, Assam'. *Indian Journal of Traditional Knowledge*, 9, 1: 52-54.

Saikia, PD. 1964. *Studies in Dafla Social and Religious Life*. Department of Tribal Culture and Folklore Research. Gauhati University.

Sajem, AL and K Gosai. 2006. 'Traditional use of medicinal plants by the Jaintia tribes in North Cachar Hill district of Assam, North East India'. *Journal of Ethno Biology and Ethnomedicine*, 2: 33.

Sharma Thakur, GC. 1999. 'Indigenous health practices and system of cure among the tribes of Assam plains', In S Sengupta (Ed.): *Health, Healers, and Healing: Studies in Medical Anthropology*. pp. 239-249. Dibrugarh; NL Publications.

Chapter - 8

Traditional Healthcare Systems among the Khamtis: A Case Study

—*Ranjumoni Hazarika*

Introduction

The word 'health' is used in the blanket form. It is generally the condition of mind and body. In recent times it is generally agreed that body and mind i.e., somatic and psychic organisations and functions are closely linked together, and there is a proximal relationship between them. At the same time, it is to be noted that the consciousness towards understanding health is seldom uniform, both in perspective of space and time. There is a great deal of variation from person to person and so based on community, gender, age group, profession, economic condition, educational background and such other attributes. Despite such variations, health is an important issue to all human beings. For all purposes, everybody wants to maintain good health. In the case of deviations, necessary care and relevant cautions are taken. It is a common understanding among the people in general that if any deviations occur in the body then it affects the other parts of the body and also the mind. It is also thought that if necessary precautions are not taken then it leads to ill health and sometimes death may occur. For such consequence, it gives rise to loss of family and also to the community and the society as a whole.

Health is practically the product of a number of systems and their operations which maintain a balance. Health can be considered as a special phenomenon of man but its existence is found to be present among almost all the members of the organic world. It is defined in many ways: World Health Organisation defines health as, '...health is a state of complete physical, mental and social well-being and not merely the absence of disease and infirmity it is, in fact, a compromise with the environment, with nature and nurture' (Polgar, 1968).

The natural environment plays an important role in the formation of tribal culture. It flourishes in specific ecological conditions. The traditional knowledge of the treatment of various diseases is a part of the tribal holistic culture. Hence the socio-cultural anthropologists take a keen interest in studying the interaction between man, society and culture in general and ethnomedicine and tribe in particular. After the trial and error method of application of herbs available in the forests, the knowledge of the same is passed on from generation to generation. This constitutes a vital aspect of folk medicine.

The concept of health and disease are basically biological. Along with these other factors like beliefs, religion, philosophy, socio-economic conditions etc also closely related to the concept of health and illness. If one considers the environmental factors of diseases than cultural factors also stand along with it. Every society has a theory of diseases and provides an efficacious for treatment. The medical treatment prevalent in a society is a combination of traditions, beliefs, techniques, ecological adaptations etc which is an integral part of the culture of the society.

Health is thus not only the interaction between an individual's hereditary contribution with his or her natural and cultural environment, but it is also largely determined by the biological and cultural adaptation and evolution of the society and the population. Health and diseases are measures of the effectiveness with which a human group has adapted to the environment. It is thus apparent that the standard of health and well-being varies with the environment, which of course varies enormously among populations or even their sub-groups.

The health of tribals depends on various factors which are inter-related to one another. The health problems of tribals stem from a double burden; the burden of health problems associated with low income, malnutrition/undernutrition, and poor sanitation and under development and other burden placed upon them by ecological/environmental changes (Tyagi, 1988). The different tribal communities have different make ups-both genetical and socio-cultural. The health of tribals depends on 'environment they live in', 'culture - including lifestyle', 'traditions and customs connected with health', 'nutrition', 'drinking water and sanitary habits', 'health and Medicare', 'diseases and indigenous Medicare' etc.

In traditional societies, people also believe in the different evil power that they consider the sources of health and illness. They believe that curse of some evil power or supernatural cause might be responsible for disturbing their normal life. To cope with such situations they take the help of medicine man.

The Khamtis at a Glance

The Khamtis are a Buddhist tribe akin to the Ahoms of Assam and belongs to the Tai linguistic group. The Tai is a generic name denoting a branch of the Mongoloid population of Asia. Within the Tai group, they are the eldest branch and so are named as Ai Tai Khamti. The majority of the Khamti are found in the southern part of Lohit district of Arunachal Pradesh. They are found scattered throughout the northern and southern banks of Brahmaputra valley in the vicinity of Sadiya region of the same river valley. To be precise the Khamtis are distributed in the foothills and plains beyond the Kamlang River and up to the southeast of the Lohit River. In the south, they have their settlements in three districts of upper Assam viz., Tinsukia, Dhemaji, and Lakhimpur. In the north, they have their settlements on the plains just below the Mishmi hills. Some of them also inhabit the Changlang district and in the north-east of Tirap district of Arunachal Pradesh-the area between Kamlang and Tirap River.

Material and Method

The data for the present study were collected from Lathao village situated 16 kilometers from Namsai main town in Lohit district in Arunachal Pradesh. The village is a homogenous one inhabited by Khamti people. The village consists of a total of 152 households and the total population is 658 out of which 400 are males and 258 are females. Data were collected through a questionnaire on types of ailments cured by the use of medicinal plants and mode of use. There was no medicinal man present in the village, but *Chao Mu* who possesses their own chants and manuscripts and have knowledge of ethnomedicine is being found to prescribe medicine or is seen performing rituals when one is found to be affected by an evil eye or any sort of supernatural factor. The *Bikkhu* of the village *Vihara* also possesses a good knowledge about the medicinal value of varieties of plants. Cross verification was also done with the respondents to see the medicine prescribed really worked or not as there was no medicine man to prescribe medicine.

Results and Discussions

The Khamtis give the least importance to their healthcare and hygiene in their normal day-to-day life especially the women folk. Their lifestyle and standard of living in the village are very simple. The food comprises of boiled sticky rice, boiled vegetables (*jabra*), boiled meat and dried fish with salt, chili and spices collected from the forests. No special recipes are prepared for children and the aged.

The dwelling houses are built on the raised platform and each family owns a hearth, and all activities are centred on the same hearth. They sit, gossip and entertain guests around the said hearth. The smoke of the hearth circulates around the kitchen and thereby affects their health, especially the eyes. The pets move freely and affect their health and even sit and sleep with them. The urinals are closely attached to their house. Due to the prevalence of such unhygienic condition, different varieties of flies and other insects breed and these subsequently become the root cause of several types of diseases of children in particular. They are not much habituated in regular bathing and changing of loin cloth. The babies are grown up in a natural course of development and also due to blessings of benevolent spirits as they believe. The mortality rate of infants is relatively more. Their style of living though has changed to some extent as the educated boys and girls take care of their health and try to maintain hygiene but the aged ones still want to cling to their traditional way of life.

Use of Medicinal Herbs and Magico-Religious Beliefs

Like other tribes, the Khamtis also have their indigenous methods of treatment of different kinds of diseases with the help of local herbal medicines. They believe that sickness and diseases are caused by malevolent spirits. There is no traditional medicine man found within the village, but *Chau Mu* is known to have some traditional knowledge of the medicinal value of plants found within the locality. The religious spiritual guide i.e., *Bhikkhus* also possess vast knowledge of ethnomedicinal plants. A number of medicinal plants are seen plants within the *Vihara* campus also.

The magico-religious practices like spirit calling ceremony form the chief antidote for most of the illness. Offerings are done, religious books are being offered in the *Vihara* as '*Danna*'. When one remains ill for a prolonged period of time, the family members approach the *Chau Mu* and he tries to identify the spirit and prescribes appropriate ritual to appease the concerned spirit. The *Chau Mu* has got its own religious texts which are totally different from Buddhist religious texts. Sometimes they perform the spirit calling ceremony commonly known as *Hong Khwon Ceremony* (*Hong* - to bring back; *Khwon*-spirit/soul) to bring back the spirit of the person. The Khamtis believe that every individual possesses a spirit within him which they call *Khwon*. So it is a spirit calling ceremony, practiced to pray the *Lengdon*-Lord of Heaven for the long life of the people.

The Khamtis believe that body and mind are governed by *Khwons* and when they are diminished, one gets affected by accidents and diseases like falling in water or from a high altitude or uncured diseases. Thus, to acquire the lost *Khwons, Hong Khwon* ceremony is performed. During this ceremony, nobody is allowed either to enter or leave the house. All the water containers are filled and household utensils are cleaned. They chant in the following way:

> 'This is the old way I am going to chant again. These have been followed by *Pu-Ching-Pha*. This is necessary for all young and old. The soul of our brother has been lost. He is becoming weak. I am going to bring back his lost soul. Then cooking pot, fish, water, bow, and arrow, spade everything is kept ready. The fishing trap is even ready. Go to a distance as much as you can cover. If you bring the soul back, the child would live long and for the whole life he would be free from illnesses.

One also approaches the religious preacher of the village *Vihar*a to consult the lunar calendar if some evil eye has caught the ill person's soul. The *Bhikkhu*, in turn, asks the family members of the patient's house to offer *Danas* in the name of the ill person, which may include their religious texts, or the *Bodhi* tree or whatever thing found by calculating the lunar calendar. He also ties the white thread in the patient's wrist by chanting *mantras*.

For treatment of minor injuries and illness, they use local herbs which are grown in abundance in their surroundings. From childhood onwards, they acquire the knowledge of identification and use of these herbal plants and this knowledge is passed on from generation to generation through experience.

The common prevalent diseases of the Khamtis of Lathao village were investigated in Lathao health centre. These include scabies, amoebiasis, helminthiasis, gastrointestinal disorder and various skin ailments along with other normal diseases like cold and cough etc. The treatment of these diseases are donc with the help of folk medicinal plants, but the acceptance rate has somewhat increased towards the use of allopathic medicines, especially the youths, for immediate relief and proper cure. They also show some interest towards Homeopathy for the treatment of chronic diseases. There are however instances of simultaneous treatment using allopathic medicines and also the performance of religious rituals conducted by *Chau Mu*.

Table 8.1: Prevalence of diseases among the patients of Lathao Village

Name of Disease	*No. of Patients*	*Percentage*	*Male*	*Female*
Fever	143	23.83	68	75
Abdomen pain	113	18.83	21	92
Chest pain	97	16.16	55	42
Scabies	82	13.66	33	49
Malaria	47	7.83	31	16
Gynecological disorder	29	4.83		29
Respiratory problem	27	4.5	13	14
Tuberculosis	23	3.83	17	6
Diarrhoea	16	2.66	14	2
Urinary infection	14	2.33	2	12
Dysentery	9	1.5	3	6
Total	**600**	**100**	**257**	**343**

(Data collected from Lathao Health Centre Register Book, 2012).

Prenatal check up during pregnancy is very rare and immunisation of babies is not considered important. It was found during case study that pregnant women reduce the amount of food intake as they believe that this would reduce the size of the foetus thus leading to a safe delivery. Maternal mortality is a bit high among the Khamtis. They prefer to give birth to children at home as they feel secure in the home. Until a few years ago colostrums was not given to the newborn baby, but nowadays it is given by the consent of medical practitioners. Though the *Asha Karmis* are there in the village, it is they who have to move from household to household in listing the pregnant women and advising them to follow the immunisation process, but the Khamti women do not take initiative in this regard. The aged person treats all the disease, in the same way, for them, all fevers are alike and hardly makes any difference between simple fever, malaria, pneumonia, viral fever etc. Likewise, he treats stomach pain in the same way whatever the cause may be.

Table 8.2: Medicinal use of plants by the Khamtis of Lathao Village

Name of Plant		*Part of Plant Used*	*Form of Medicine*	*Disease*
Local Name	*Botanical Name*			
Mak Khom	*Phyllanthus embilca*	fruit	Powder of the fruit (dry)	1. Used during constipation

(Cont'd...)

Tun tonh kou	*Musa balbisinia*	inflorescence	Soup of the inflorescence	1. Given to the new mother so that more milk develops.
Tun puthi kham	*Punica grantam*	the twig	juice extract	1. Stop excessive bleeding during pregnancy. 2. irregular menstruation
Tun rung rai/hai	*Ficus religiosa*	Bark and	Paste is mixed tender roots	1. Curing of contagious disease of genital organ. 2. White discharge of women.
Linfaa	*Azadirachata indica*	Leaf, bark	The extracted water after boiling the leaf/twig	1. Skin diseases 2. Constipation
Man na domestica	*Curcuma*	rhizomes	The paste and juice	1. applied to that part when one gets hurt
Pan na	*Terminalia*	The fruit	Paste is mixed with salt	1. piles 2. constipation 3. acidity *chebula* or roots
Tun mai pu mum	*Terminalia bellirica*	The fruit, the roots	Paste of root mixed with a pinch of salt and filtered water	1. white discharge of women 2. gastro-intestinal disorders 3. treating asthma 4. sore throat
Mak lang pha	*Annona reticulata* and barks	Fragments of roots is boiled	Paste of roots bark 2. in water	1. packed around the gums to relieve a toothache bark serve as a tonic to diarrhoea and dysentery
Mak pokna	*Aegele marmelos* unripe fruit pulp	Leaves and	decoction	1. treat cholera 2. diabetes 3. jaundice Also, decoction of aegele, neem and juice of tulsi is used to decrease symptoms of HIV/AIDS
Mak lang pha	*Annona squamosa*	Unripe fruit	Boiled in water in case of small children	1. cure diarrhoea 2. dysentery
Khum phat	*Bischofia javanica*	roots	Decoction	1. Cure diarrhoea
Mak mip meo	*Flacourtia*	Fruits, leaves, young shoots and bark	decoction	1. stomach pain 2. digestion 3. relief from nausea 4. leaves are used in diarrhoea, piles 5. bark decoction in a toothache and bleeding gums
Mak pha kham	*Phyllanthus acidus*	Fruit,	Decoction in	1. emetic and purgative 2. used in respiratory problem

(*Cont'd...*)

				3. skin diseases 4. bronchitis 5. sores 6. coughs
Blok theng	*Mesua ferrea*	Seeds and flowers	Oil is extracted	1. Oil extracted from seeds is used in antifungal activity against a number of pathogenic fungi. 2. Oil from flowers is used against antibacterial activity 3. Curing of skin ailments
Tun-oo-nu-cha	*Nyctanthes arbortristris*	Flowers, stem, leaves	decoction	1. flowers are used for ophthalmic purposes, used as hair tonic and treatment of piles 2. stem is powdered and used in joint pain 3. bark is used against snakebite and treatment of malaria 4. Leaves are used in a cough, piles, chronic fever and intestinal worms.
Mak thap	*Borassus flabellifer*	Leaf, flower stalks	Decoction, juice extraction from leaves	1. decoction of the fibrous fruit is used for gonorrhea and respiratory ailments 2. leaf juice is used for gastric ailments 3. base of leaves is used for external wounds 4. Juice from flowering stalks is used for diabetes.

Conclusion

Though the tendency towards modern treatment has gradually increased, yet the use of ethnomedicine is still prevalent among the villagers. Though manifold modern medical facilities are being provided, it has come to light that a large number of people still depend on indigenous medical treatment. The *Chau Mu* still plays a major role in diagnosis as well as the application of medicine and performing the rituals for relief from the sufferings. Though there is a change in the attitude of the Khamtis of Lathao village in respect of certain traditional concepts and practices persist in the presence of modern health services and irrespective of the degree of health facilities.

References

Polgar, S. 1968. 'Health'. In DL. Sills (Ed): *International Encyclopedia of the Social Sciences,* New York; Mcmillar and Free Press.

Singh, BK, 2008. *Encyclopaedia of Ai Tai Khamti*, Chaukham; Chow Meohou Namchoom.

Tyagi, D., 1988. 'Tribal population and health', *Paper presented in Tribal Situation in India,* organised by Ethnographic and Folk Culture Society and State Planning Commission, Lucknow.

W.H.O., 1964. *Human Genetic and Public Health*, Tech. Report. Serial Number 282, Geneva.

Chapter - 9

Use of Indigenous Plants in Traditional Healthcare Systems among the Mishing Tribe of Assam

—*Ratna Jyoti Das*

Introduction

The Mishing (Miri) is an Indo-Mongoloid and East Asian group of people migrated from the eastern Himalayan regions in Tibet in the hoary past and finally settled in the fertile Brahmaputra valley in Assam province of India. While migrating to Assam, the Mishing followed mainly the course of the Brahmaputra, gradually spreading to other stretches of land lying on the banks of its tributaries like the Dihing, Disang, Dikhow, the Subansiri, the Ranganadi, the Dikrong, etc. with habitations scattered now in eight districts of the state, viz. Tinsukia, Dibrugarh, Dhemaji, Lakhimpur, Sibsager, Jorhat, Golaghat and Sonitpur. Dikhowmukh is the place where Dikhow River is joining to the Brahmaputra River in Sivasagar district. On the bank of both Dikhow River and Brahmaputra river of Dikhowmukh village, Mishing tribes are residing since a long time ago.

The Mishings are known to use a good number of wild plants as traditional food and folklore medicines (Barua *et al.*, 2007). The Mishings with their rich cultures contributes to the cultural diversity of the region. It is generally seen that the Mishing women play a very significant role in the society. They are also known to be highly passionate about cooking traditionally unique food items as well as for various folklore medicines (Barua *et al.*, 2007). Hence, the elderly Mishing women are like a store house of various information and could be used as a source for many important traditional knowledge systems of the community (Kohli, 2001).

The present study was carried out to enlist the indigenous plant species used as folklore medicine for treatment of certain ailments and also as traditional food having possible medicinal values (Neog and Mohan, 1994; Saikia and Shadeque, 1993).

Materials and Methods

Assam is one of the Indian states with 2.8 percent of the total area of the Indian Union and 2.7 percent of its population. It is located between 90^0 -96^0 East longitudes and 22^0-26^0 north latitude. Sivasagar district is extended between $26^0 45'$ - $27^0 15'$ N latitude and $94^0 25'$ -$95^0 25'$ E longitude. The study was carried out in Dikhowmukh village of Sivasagar district. Dikhowmukh village is approximately 23 km away from Sivasagar town. The study area is under Sivasagar subdivision. The average annual rainfall is 108.44 cm and temperature varies in between 15^0 to 35^0 c

The study was conducted through extensive personal interviews, in-depth discussions and participant observations with the traditional medical practitioners and selected knowledge holders of Mishing tribe of Dikhowmukh villages in Sivasagar district, Assam. The target groups of the present study comprise elderly persons both male and female of the Mishing tribal community above 40 years, who practices the traditional healthcare systems. Some of them are folk healers and some are not. They are usually cultivators and most of them are familiar with the traditional uses of indigenous plants in various purposes. Moreover, the housewives who collect different wild plants as vegetables for cooking purposes were also considered for an interview.

The questionnaires were prepared to get the direct information on the traditional knowledge that is prevailing and usually practiced in the community. The indigenous plant species used by the Mishing tribe were collected from the field as shown by the respondents and the detail information about the plants and parts used in the treatment of different ailments were collected. Most of the plants were commonly occurring plants and known to most of the people. All the enumerated plant species were identified with the help of relevant and standard literature (Dutta, 1985; Gupta and Sharma, 2007, 2008).

Results and Discussions

During the present study, 12 different plant species were found to use as traditional healthcare services by the village Mishing people of Dikhowmukh, Sivasagar district. Table 9.1 enlists the indigenous plant species commonly used by the Mishing tribe of the study area. Though people of the study areas access to the healthcare services, yet they prefer folklore medicines for certain ailments as immediate and effective measures

(Saikia and Hussain, 2004). Both male and female were found to possess good knowledge of folklore medicines specially derived from plants (Table 9.1). The habits of using forest-based wild herbs, shrubs, climbers, and trees for cooking purposes are unique to the Mishing tribe. The recent trends of habitat destruction and decrease in the forest area has rendered many species to disappear from the environment for which household of the Mishing tribal community is maintaining some easily propagatable of frequently used plant species such as *D. wallichiana, N. feylavica, F. glomerata, Z. hamiltonianum* etc. in the backyard of their house in order to achieve their immediate needs.

Table 9.1: Indigenous plant species commonly used by the Mishing tribe

Sl. no	*Scientific name*	*Local name in Assamese*	*Family*	*Parts used*	*Uses*
1	*Mimosa pudica* L.	*Nilaji*	Mimosaceae	Root	Tooth worm, Menstrual problem
2	*Hydrocotyle rotundifolia* Roxb.	*Horu manimuni*	Apicaeae	Leaves, Roots	Dysentery, diarrhea, piles, rheumatism, as digestive, diuretic and vermifuge and menstrual problem
3	*Bambusa balcooa* Roxb	*Bholuka bah*	Poaceae	Shoots,	Painkiller in insect bites and menstrual problem Young leaves
4	*Caesalpinia crista* Linn.	*Leta Guti*	Caesal-pinaceae		Fruits Used with *D. cordata* in fever and fruits are used as a tonic and antipyretic.
5	*Leucas aspera* Spreng	*Durun bon*	Lamiaceae	Leaves, Root	Leaves are used in lack of appetite, Sinusitis, stomach complaints, and headache. The leaf extract is used in skin problems. Roots are used to treat pneumonia, swellings, ringworms, boils etc and in the relief of snake bites.
6	*Musa balbisiana* Colla	*Bhim kol*	Musaceae	Fruit, Root	Stomach problems and dys entery. Roots are used to treat pneumonia
7	*Piper nigrum* Linn.	*Jaluk*	Piperaceae	Fruits	The fruits are consumed in indigestion, body-ache and in the post labour ailment and in bone fractures and pneumonia
8	*Eichornia crassipes Solams*	*Meteka*	Ponte-deriaceae	Flowers/ roots	Stomach ache/ trouble, roots are used in the treat-ment of pneumoni

(*Cont'd...*)

9	*Cordia dichotoma*	*Buwal*	Boraginaceae	Bark	Stomach problem, gastritis
10	*Nyctanthes arbor tristis*	*Khewali*	Oleaceae	Leaves	Cutting wounds, to stop bleeding
11	*Pachystachys lutea*	*Hunboronia*	Acanthaceae	Root	To treat pneumonia
12	*Adhatuda vesica*	*Bosa*	Acanthaceae	Root	To treat pneumonia, chest affections, expectorant, bronchitis, asthma, tuberculosis, diarrhoea, dysentery, and malaria.

From the study, it was found that among 12 different plants used as indigenous plants by the Mishing tribe of the study area, six plants are mainly used for the treatment of Pneumonia. Those plants are namely, *Leucas aspera* Spreng, *Musa balbisiana* Colla, *Piper nigrum* Linn. *Eichornia crassipes* Solams, *Pachystachys lutea,* and *Adhatuda vesica.* One method of treatment of Pneumonia is given in formula 1.

Formula 1

Plant	***Part***	***Quantity***
Pachystachys lutea	Root	1 plant
Piper nigrum	Seed	3-4 no
Leucas aspera spreng	Root	1 plant

All parts were ground together and a small amount of water is added. The juice part is separated and salt is to be added and finally, the dosage form is ready to be used.

Like other tribal communities, the Mishing of Dikhowmukh village also has deep faith in the efficacy of incantation (*mantras*) in curing diseases. Traditional healer (*Bej*) will diagnose the cause of the illness through divination. At the time of divination, he will invoke the dead ancestors and Gods, through appropriate spells and incantations. They will convey the causes and remedies of illness to the *Bej* and he will treat the patient according to these directions. According to a *Bej* of Mishing tribe, there are four major causes of illness; namely, (i) anger of God, (ii) anger of ancestral spirits, (iii) breach of taboo and (iv) possession of evil spirits. The traditional mantras still hold an important place in the Mishing society. The villagers are using these traditional mantras for the treatment of diseases like the pain of chest, feet, and other parts of the body, snakebite, tonsillitis, piles, bleeding of women, etc. In the Mishing society, apart from the local medicine men who treat most of the diseases, one comes across other specialists in bone-setting, curing of a bite by dog, fox and snake and healing of burn injuries. All of them are known as *Bej* in their society. The *Bejs* are ordinary cultivators or even landless labourers. They are generally males and their posts are not hereditary. Women are not permitted to be a *bej* because of their patriarchy nature. The *Bej* accepts remuneration in the form of a feast if the patient gets cured. The bulk of the drugs used by the *Bejs* to cure prevalent diseases is of vegetable origin. Apart from oral consumption of herbals certain other forms of treatment such as bathing, fumigation, fomentation, application of purgative, etc. are in vogue.

Conclusion

A deep-rooted indigenous bio-cultural heritage surrounding plant resource utilisation forms an inseparable part of the life of the Mishing tribe of Assam. The present chapter is an effort made to explore and document some vital aspects of the plant based traditional skills and technologies related to ethnomedicine and consumption of wild edible plants by the Mishing people of Dikhowmukh village, Sivasagar. Further scientific research on the plant based indigenous knowledge can provide ample scope for further pharmaceutical studies as well as in the development of eco-friendly technologies for better livelihood.

References

Barua, U., DK. Hore and R. Sarma. 2007. 'Wild edible plants of Majuli island and Darang districts of Assam', *Indian Journal of Traditional Knowledge*, 6, 1: 191-194.

Dutta, AC., 1985. *Dictionary of Economic and Medicinal Plants*, Khelmati, Jorhat, Assam.

Gupta, AK and M. Sharma, 2007. *Reviews on Indian Medicinal Plants*, Vol. V, New Delhi; Medicinal Plant Unit, ICMR.

Gupta, AK and M. Sharma, 2008. *Reviews on Indian Medicinal Plants*, Vol. VI, New Delhi; Medicinal Plant Unit, ICMR.

Kohli, YP., 2001. 'Non-traditional foods and ethnobotanical plants of lower Subansiri district, Arunachal Pradesh', *Arunachal Forest News*, 19, 1-2:169-171.

Neog, M, and HK. Mohan, 1994. 'Minor and less known fruits of Assam', *Indian Horticulture,* 39: 28-31.

Saikia, A and A. Shadeque, 1993. 'Nutritional evaluation of under-exploited leafy vegetables of Assam', *Indian Journal of Agricultural Science*, 63: 409-411.

Saikia, LR, and I. Hussain, 2004. 'Indigenous fruits used as folklore medicine by Ahom and Khamti communities of Sivasagar district', *National Journal of Life Sciences,* 2, 1: 389-394.

Chapter - 10

The Role of Folk Medical Practitioners During and after Flood: A Case Study of Mishing Medical Practitioners of Dhemaji District

—Dipa Patir Changmai and Dharmendra Changmai

Introduction

Folk medicine has existed for as long as human beings have existed. In an effort to cope with an environment that was often dangerous, humans, and their ancestors began to develop ways of lessening pain and treating physical and mental problems. At first, many of the ways of treating these problems undoubtedly came through trial and error methods, using various plants and other methods derived from observation of how animals reacted to and treated illnesses and injuries. Over time, individuals within family and tribal groups became more skilled at helping the sick and injured, and some of them became responsible for carrying out healing ceremonies, religious rituals, and other rites designed to ensure the safety and health of their communities. However, the tribal people were great believers of folk medicine.

The anthropologists generally see the field of primitive medicines in two main aspects (i) as a cultural complex, i.e., complex of material objects, tools, techniques, knowledge of indigenous leaves, plants, ideas and values and (ii) as a part of social structure i.e., a network of relations between group, clans and categories of persons. In both these aspects the anthropologists are interested in medicine; especially the indigenous medicines which are being practiced by the tribal people as knowledge of the indigenous medicinal plants influence the socio-religious life of the tribal society.

In many tribal societies, various types of plants and leaves are used to get rid of disease/ wounds, etc., and those who are specialised in this treatment are accorded high status in the societies.

A folk healer is an unlicensed person who practices the art of healing using traditional practices, herbal remedies and even the power of suggestion. A folk healer may be a highly trained person who pursues his specialties, learning by observation and imitation. In some cultures, a healer might be considered to be a person who has inherited the 'gift' of healing from his or her parent. The ability to set bones or the power to stop bleeding may be thought of as hereditary powers.

The folk medical practitioner or traditional healer can be defined as 'someone who is recognised by the community in which he lives as competent to provide healthcare by using vegetable, animal and mineral substances and certain other methods based on the social, cultural and religious backgrounds as well as the prevailing knowledge, attitudes and beliefs regarding physical, mental and social well-being and the causation of disease and disability in the community'. Traditional healers used different medicinal formulae from various natural substances (animal, mineral and vegetable). They have extensive knowledge on the use of plants and herbs for medicinal and nutritional purposes.

The Mishing people, due to their habitation close to river banks are susceptible to malaria and water-borne diseases and for which they could develop traditional healing practices to protect themselves from different diseases since time immemorial. Traditional healing practices of those days are still preferred by the people of this community in this modern era.

Traditional healing practices amongst Mishing tribe is the method to treat ailments by using herbs in the form of freshly crushed juice, decoction of drug part and powdered medicine for oral intake and paste for local application on skin diseases and wounds. They use locally available medicinal herbs, cultivated medicinal plants from different habitat as well as cultivating depleting medicinal plants. They have also faith on divine power and worships nature for the cure of ailments. The study entails detailed documentation of healing practices used by traditional healers for their community health with full faith and confidence. Malaria and jaundice are the prominent diseases in North East India which are caused during and after the flood and are widely treated by traditional healers. Around 68 herbs have been recorded treating malaria and about 88 for treating jaundice.

Assam is situated in the north-eastern region of India lying between 24°- 28° N and 90°- 96° E. The entire northeastern region comprises eight states (Assam, Arunachal Pradesh, Manipur, Meghalaya, Nagaland, Tripura, Mizoram, and Sikkim). North East India with its rich floristic diversity is also inhabited by the largest number of tribes and they lead an intricate life totally dependent on the forest plants. The overall tribal population of this region accounts for more than 57 per cent of the total population. In Assam alone, the percentage of the tribal population is 12.83. More than 25 communities, mostly tribal and mainly depending on plant resources for their day-to-day life inhabit in the different parts of the state. They have a close association with and good knowledge about plant resources of their surroundings which form an integral part of their material and spiritual cultures.

The Mishing with a population of 6,80,424 (as per 2011 census), constitute the second largest plains Scheduled Tribe of Assam. The settlement areas of the tribe under study are chiefly Dhemaji, Lakhimpur, Dibrugarh, Tinsukia, Sibsagar, Sonitpur, Darang, Jorhat and Golaghat districts of Assam.

By faith, they are the worshippers of '*Dony*' (the Sun) and '*Polo*' (the Moon). They claim themselves as the children of nature. They perform a number of religious practices in their life. The practices are comprised of various rites and rituals of prayer, offerings, and sacrifices. They believe that after death the spirits which they call *'Uie*' roam invisibly around them and these *Uies* are always hostile to human beings. Generally, the spirits causing troubles are diagnosed by the '*Mibu*' (Mishing priest).

Role of folk medical practitioners during and after flood

During the course of study, traditional healers were interviewed from Sissiborgaon block of Dhemaji district. They were Mrs. K. K. age 70 years of Borkuli village of Kulajan; Mr. B. P. age 82 years of Tanteri village of Kulajan; and Mr. K. P. age 81 years of Patgiri gaon. Detail information about the plants used in the treatment of different ailments was collected as given by folk practitioners. The knowledge of the use of plants has descended down traditionally i.e. it has been transferred from one generation to other without any documentation and some of the curative folk medicine has been learned from the nearby community. Now they are expert folk medical practitioners of their localities. When we interviewed Mr. B. P. asking him about the treatment of jaundice, he said that 'jaundice mainly appears during the summer season and it mostly appears in flood affected areas. In our localities the villagers do not go to the doctor, they bring their patients to my house; and if the patient is serious they call me to their house'. He gives some home remedy to cure the diseases which are made from the bark of mango tree (*Mangifera indica*), one fist of *lai juburi* (*Drymaria cordata*) and a small quantity of lime.

The extract (about 50 gm) mixed with water is given to take in the empty stomach on an alternate day and after 10 minutes the patients can take their meal. The patient has to take three *pali* (dose) and for the serious patient, it may be up to six *pali* (dose). There is some restriction of food which patients have to follow; they have to avoid foods like, meat, fish, potato, oil, spicy and any other fatty items. The patients are also advised to eat only boil items especially boiled green vegetables.

According to Mrs. K. K. of Borkuli village, 'traditional healing practiced by us is the method to treat ailments by using herbs in the form of freshly crushed juice, decoction of drug part and powdered medicine for oral intake and paste for local application on skin diseases and wounds. I use locally available medicinal herbs, cultivated in different habitat as well as by cultivating the rare medicinal plants. The treatments of diseases which I commonly render are diarrhea, tonsil, seasonal pox, complicacy during delivery, tumor, stone problem etc. Diarrhea, tonsil, fever, seasonal pox, are common in our area due to annual flood. During the flood, some delivery cases are also consulted with me by the family members because at that time the villagers mostly remain disconnected from the available health resources'.

Methodology of the Treatment

When the patient suffers from diarrhea, a mixture of juice of banana locally called *aathia kopak* (*Musa bulbisiana*) and juice of crushed guava leaves locally called *muduri anne* (*Psidium guava*) is offered to the patient. And for respiratory infections such as common cold and mild flu, chicken soup (decoction of chicken, black pepper, turmeric, *marsang*, *pipali pat*, salt, and *bilongoni*) is given to the patient. For tonsil treatment the mixture of maize seed powder, cloves, locally called *laung* (*Syzygium aromaticum*), nut-meg - local name *Jaifol* (*Myristica fragrans*), wild black pepper locally called *bon jaluk* (*Oldenlandia corymbosa*) are mixed with honey, after that, the mixture is given to the patient for seven days to reduce infection. For seasonal pox, the mixture of crushed juice of Indian pennywort local name *bunki repuk*, Assamese name *manimuni* (*Centella asiatica*), and sugar candy locally called *misiri*, and *mosondori* (*Houttuynia cordata*) is given to take orally.

If the complicacy appears during delivery, the traditional healer (Mrs K. K.) used to take a root of arum plant, locally called *enge* (*Colocasia esculenta*) and prays her *guru*, after that she tie the arum root in the patients' neck in a single breathes.

Folk medicines used by Mr. K. P., a traditional healer of Patgiri village to cure disease, during and after the flood, like diarrhea, malaria, skin disease like ringworm and Whitlow etc. For diarrhea treatment bark of *bangee* tree and powder of *Hilikha* seed (*Terminali chebula*) is boiled for 20 minutes in 500 ml water, the decoction of 50 ml is given thrice daily for three days. *Hilika* plants used to cure malaria are 50 gm of the bark of a *bangee* tree, *Sirota* (*Swertia chirayita*), *Hewali* leaf (*Nyetanthes abor-tristis*), the bark of *Satiana* tree (*Alstonia Scholaris*) and *Tulsi* leaf (*Ocimum sanctum*). These are boiled in a pan and the decoction of 50 ml is given twice daily for three days.

To cure the skin disease like ringworm the plant he (Mr K. P.) used is *khar pat* (*Cassia alata*). The number of *Khar pat* should be used in odd numbers for example 1, 3, 5 etc. and at the time of plucking no one should look him. The affected part is washed with lukewarm water and then the paste of leaves is applied on it. There is another method by which one can cure the same disease. For this method, child stool is applied on the affected area and rubbed by a coin taken from the infected person.

Treatment of Snake

During the flood in some area of Sissi Borgaon block, the water level comes above the platform and that time snake and other ants come out with water and enter into the villager's house and bite someone. When a person is bitten by a snake, firstly the local healer used to tie with a long hair of female at the bitten spot. After that, the traditional healer placed the chicken anus just on the bite spot to suck out the poison. After repeating the process several times the chicken will die due to sucking of poison. And again another chicken is placed on the spot as before. If this time the chicken does not die, healer announces that there is no more poison left in the patient.

Practice of ordeal to reduce complicacy

The practice of ordeal is still found in some places of Mishing community. When we went to Jonai to meet a '*myibu*' (shamanist priest possessing some supernatural power and knowledge that performs the traditional and religious rituals) named Tulsi Pegu, he told us about the practice of ordeal which is still seen in their community during delivery of a pregnant woman and the knowledge of serving different treatment of different ailments. In some place in their community if a pregnant woman had done any sin enjoying sex with a prohibited person, then she gets problems during child delivery or becomes very complicated and in this case, they adopted various means to make the easy delivery. At the first stage of complicacy, a '*myibu*' (shamanist priest possessing some supernatural power) is called who through divination with the help of egg or chicken liver tries to find out the spirit with sacrifices of a chick or a fowl or a cork, pig or so. Even after the performance of the prescribed remedies if the delivery does not occur she is pressurised by some ladies if she had any illicit relation before, or even after her marriage. In such case, the woman in labour pain is frightened and usually comes out with the confession of her past sin. If she afraid to confess her sin then the husband is asked to put his great toe into the water in a pot and that water are given to his wife to drink. After that, a piece of cloth is taken out from her husband's underwear and ties it around her waist and applies mustard oil to her lower abdomen. If it is a case of *myibu* then he takes resort to supernatural means for delivery of the baby. He makes a thread with the special colour combination, chants spell on it, and then making it like a necklace gives the woman in labour pain to put on. Such a garland sort of things is to be put on her neck. The spell chanted in the threads lends some elasticity to it. For, after the putting on it, if the case remains still complicated, the threads get lengthened so much so that the garland like thread passes through the whole body of the lady and ultimately it falls on the ground. To their belief with the fall of the thread ring from the lady's body the baby also fall on the ground.

The traditional healers diagnose the ailments with the help of "*dogne*"-precious and spiritual beads which contains divine power and with the help of "*yoksa*", a potent sword having celestial power.

Conclusion

The study on the role of folk medical practitioners of Mishing community during and after the flood in Dhemaji district of Assam was made to document the healing practices used by the Mishing community with details of methodology and doses. To cope up with the problems the villagers still believe on the local folk medical practitioners. These practitioners are the first to be consulted when a family member becomes ill. Prevalent diseases treated by the Mishing healers are Jaundice, malaria, fever, skin diseases etc.

Presently all traditional healers of the community are not performing the same functions, nor do they all fall into the same category. Each of them has their own field of expertise. Even the techniques employed differed considerably. They have their own methods of diagnosis and their own particular medicine. It is also noticed that in some places of Mishing community practice of ordeal is still found which is not a good sign for Mishing woman.

References

Nath, J, and NK. Pegu, 2012. *A Cultural History of the Mishing of Assam*. Guwahati; Prithibi Prakashan.

Shankar, R.; GS. Lavekar; S. Deb and BK. Sharma, 2012. 'Traditional healing practice and folk medicines used by Mishing community of North East India'. *Journal of Ayurveda Integrative Medicine*, 3:124-129.

Sharma, UK and S. Pegu, 2011. 'Ethnobotany of religious and supernatural beliefs of the Mishing tribe of Assam with special reference to the *Dobur Uei*'. *Journal of Ethnobiology and Ethnomedicine* 7: 16.

Taye, N., 2009. *Sirki Nane. A Religious Culture and Traditional North-East India, Assam and Arunachal Pradesh,* Guwahati; Rajdhani Offset, www.assamplants.com

Chapter - 11

Child Rearing Practices among the Mishings of Assam

—*Mondira Boruah*

Introduction

Children are considered as the most valuable asset of the nation, they are the future citizen and the nation builders. To be a good citizen an individual requires inculcating good personality and habits that depend on its foundation period childhood. Hence, development of a nation always reflects how its children's are being cared and brought up. A family where the child belongs to is the basic unit of the society. Each and every family has to follow certain norms and rules of the particular society to get recognition and identity. In other words, every society has its traditionally and culturally practiced norms and upbringing of its children. Home is the primary institute of child rearing, the term child-rearing is considered as the upbringing of children in a family with all interactions among parents, interests, beliefs, caretaking and training behaviour to make their children the acceptable member of the society.

Studies conducted on various aspects of child rearing have been relied on to supplement and sharpen the various stages of this study. The classic work on child rearing practices was done by Mead in 1963. It is seen that studies related to child rearing are very few and those on tribes of the North East are even very fewer. Here an attempt has been made to review the relevant studies conducted on the various aspects of child rearing practices. Rajani *et al.* (1979:317-319) studied on existing sex ratio and impact of family planning on sex ratio in Visakhapatnam, Andhra Pradesh. Sharma and Khan (1990:446-453) found that the Khariwar tribal women exhibit 4.85 live births per mother and 145 infant deaths per thousand live births. The researchers observed that lack of medical facilities and their worst environmental conditions were the attributed causes of high mortality and morbidity rates. Muthal (1992: 97-103) studied on attitudes towards fertility control. He founds that higher income and higher educational level, to a large extent are responsible for changes in beliefs and attitudes towards adopting modern attitudes towards fertility control. Srivastava (1971: 182-183) found that pregnant mothers of Asalpur (Rajasthan) and Barigaon (Uttar Pradesh) at their advanced stages of pregnancies they are not allowed to lift a heavy weight, they also avoid places believed to be haunted by evil spirits, crossing a river is also tabooed for them during pregnancy.

Bhuyan (1993:81-95) studied among the four tribes of Assam and observed that total 29 per cent of the respondents follow certain dietary restrictions during pregnancy. The Tai Khamiyangs of Assam used to bury the placenta within the compound and they never give any pressure on it and it is also found among the Mao and Kabui tribes of Manipur. Some worth mentioning studies on child rearing are done by Dastidhar and Gupta (1996:63-69), NIPCCS (1998:75), Boruah and Bora (1999:336), Sinha and Pandey (2000:338-339), Tribhuwan and Gambhir (2001:4-7).

The present study is concerned about the child-rearing practices among the Mishings of Dhemaji district of Assam. The study is based on a study of total 35 households of the village Bongalmari of Dhemaji district. The main objective of the study is to find out the process of child rearing practices, and health and hygiene of the children of age group up to nine months. The study will focus on the relationship between the family and the child, the process of socialisation, the basic disciplines, practices and process of child rearing, health and hygiene practices related to child and the home remedies etc. The study is based on the primary and secondary data. The methods used to collect primary data are observation, case study, survey schedule and in-depth interviews in this study.

Amongst all mammals, the human being is born as the most dependent creatures from all aspects. It needs all types of physical and mental care and protection. It also born with most educable nature, which can be molded as desired to give a particular shape. As mentioned above the adult personality is formed on its foundation child rearing.Though different psychologists and educationalists have defined childhood period in terms of years /age variedly, they all agreed to it that this period is a most crucial one, which later forms adult personality. It would be a misconception of child rearing if we consider overall care of a child only after birth. Since proper growth and development of a child depend on its health status at birth and as it is very closely associated with its prenatal and natal period, hence care during these periods also assumes importance. Direct care cannot be given to the child during the prenatal period and it depends completely on its mother, therefore care of mother in all aspects is very necessary. Child rearing, therefore, encompasses care of the mother during pregnancy and postpartum period including nutritional and healthcare, sleep, and rest, care of the newborn and young children, such as breastfeeding, weaning, complementary feeding, healthcare, toilet training recreation etc. Child rearing practices basically take into account the following four aspects:

Family and child: After birth, in the very beginning of human life, generally the mother is considered as the basic trainer of the child in the family, later the family members and ultimately the society. Since the family is the best workshop for the child; he should be given adequate opportunity to stimulate his responses; so that the child can adjust himself to the new environment. Although in all families the young ones are fed protected, nursed, dependency needs are attended, yet the child rearing practices are not alike everywhere cultural factors have great influence on children since they are deeply rooted in the socialisation of children. When a child is born, it enters into such an environment, which surrounded, by a number of cultural laws and rules of the society and parents want to give all the bests to their children within their affordability. All methods knowingly or unknowingly adopted by the parents to rear their children may not be socialistically acceptable. There are certain specific activities, which need special attention of parents in order to regulate and control the milestone of the development of their children in a wholesome way (Panda, 1990: 93).

Socialisation: The term socialisation refers to the process by which the child is being prepared to be a member of the society. Each society is fabricated by its own cultural traits, motives, values, rules, and code of conduct. The child has to proceed through all these to be an acceptable member of the society. By socialisation, the child is trained about the norms and rules of the society and he or she acquires the attitudes and values of that culture to adjust in that socio-cultural environment, with culturally approved behaviour. Discipline is a practical problem of child rearing by which the child is prepared to make himself an adequate adult member of the society to which he belongs. There is a very close relationship between the prenatal practices in the upbringing of children and the behaviour pattern of adults. There are two ways in which unique types of thinking feeling and mode of acting of a particular group of people transmitted to the next generation, first directly and formally, second informally.

The basic disciplines: Primarily the term discipline refers is to control especially over the undesirable behaviour of children. In other sense, it is any kind of influence designed to help the child to learn the socially approved behaviours. Discipline does not mean giving punishment and imply of strict rules on children. The three main elements of discipline are education, reward, and punishment. By birth, the child does not come with the sense of judging behaviour that is socially approved or disapproved. This tender human bud needs to be trained with great care, blending the three features of discipline in the right proportion and a correct age. Rules in educating or training the child are essential because they acquaint the child with standards of conduct acceptable to the group and they restrain undesirable behaviour (Kuppuswami, 1980; 186). Likewise giving reward or praising the child is very important, because it promotes and facilitates learning through brightening and contributing healthy emotional growth. Punishment in discipline is necessary to make the child understand about the misbehaving that he or she did. However, both reward and punishment need to be understood by the child, otherwise, it will be wasted. There must be one objective of giving reward or punishment and should be explained to the child, otherwise, the child will be lost in confusion.

Child rearing practices: The child rearing practices include everything from the period of conception. The reproductive health of the women generally confines to the female reproductive organs and is particularly, relating to childbearing. It begins at the time of onset of menarche and continues till the women attain menopause. The concept of reproductive health was first developed by World Health Organisation. Later, WHO's definition retreated at the international reproductive health measures. Reproductive health thus implies that women can go safely through pregnancy and childbirth. For proper growth, development of the baby mother's health plays a very crucial role. Babies' life after birth is very closely linked with its life in mother's womb, only a healthy mother can produce a healthy baby. It is very necessary to make important care of the expectant mother.

When we talk about care of mother in child rearing, it includes three aspects, namely antenatal, natal care, and postnatal care. Antenatal care is children's regular health check up by medicine practitioners and proper work, rest, and exercise to the expectant mother. The natal care consists the process of delivery by trained birth attendant use of safety equipment, cleanliness etc. And postnatal care is a health check up, diet, rest etc to the child and the mother. The care of the mothers in these three periods greatly influence for the survival of the child, for its growth and development and general well being. The maternity care has a direct relationship with the babies' health and growth.

Besides these medical cares, in a society, a pregnant woman with her baby has to follow some rules and regulations governed by the society. Being an integral part of the society mother is surrounded by numbers of traditional beliefs and superstition with one without reason simply has to obey and follow these beliefs and restrictions. The fetus inside the mother's womb is completely dependent on its mother. The growth and development of the foetus will be satisfactory if the expectant mother is given proper dietary attention, in many societies performance of rites for proper delivery is common everywhere. A successful delivery reduces the mortality morbidity both the child and the mother.

After the birth of the baby, important care should be taken to the baby. The human newborn is perhaps the most delicate one amongst all living beings in the world. The helpless neonate needs all types of care to be adjusted in the new environment. By birth when there is a transition from intrauterine to extrauterine life the newborn is exposed to external temperature and environment certain functions of the baby involving the lungs, central nervous system, digestion, endocrinal, immunological maintenance of body temperature etc taken place independently.

Immediate newborn care including cleaning and bathing of the baby is very crucial and thus the newborn should be handled with great gentleness and care. These also reduce many infections and chances of life expectancy to a large extent. The newborn even die if the baby is deprived of proper care and favourable environment. Such immediate newborn care includes resuscitation. The neonate needs food, by nature, mother's milk is the most prestigious gift to the neonate. Being the principal source of nourishment it is a well-balanced food, consisting of all the necessary nutrients required for the baby. Besides mother's milk, pre-lacteal food is also given to the child. The term pre-lacteal feed denotes the food introduced to the baby before giving mother's milk. These pre-lacteal feeds are generally given to the babies who are delayed to put into the breast. It is also given in many societies even through breastfeeding is not delayed. The care of the navel is very important to save the child from, neonatal tetanus, a dreadful infection with high mortality rate. Infection usually occurs if the delivery is conducted in an unhygienic environment, an instrument used for cutting umbilical cord is dirty and unsterilised and if the naval is treated with some germ carrying materials. The bed for the newborn should usually be soft, comfortable and clean. Most of the mothers generally used old cotton clothes for making the bed for the baby. During this course, the child has learned toilet training, after one year or two years weaning started by every mother to their children. The term weaning refers to the process by which the baby is changed from its milky diet to other mixed solid diet after the sixth month of the baby mother's milk cannot give complete nourishment as the baby grows rapidly at this stage and it needs proper nourishment to attain its maximum growth. Thus, it becomes necessary to introduce other complementary foods in addition to another's milk.

The Mishings

The Mishings are also known as the Miri, but they prefer to be called by the former. The term 'Miri' is said to have been given by the Assamese of the Brahmaputra valley. This term 'Miri' as found in many old Assamese records is also found in the Vaishnavite religious scriptures.

The word Mishing connotes two syllables, namely, '*Mi*' and '*Asi*', the former 'man' and the letter, 'water', that is, the people in some way or other are in constant touch with water, meaning a source of water, so it means the people live in the riverside areas (Baruah, 2010: 44-45). The colourful ethnic group living amidst of the fellow Assamese people is the second largest group of Scheduled Tribe (plains) of Assam. It is a truism that the Mishings, originally a hill tribe within the ranges of Abor, Miri and Mishing hills of the erstwhile North East Frontier Agency now Arunachal Pradesh and they came down to the plains before the reign of the Ahom Kingdom. The ethnic group is very rich with their own cultural aspects, such as dialect, rules, and regulations, religious beliefs, festivals, material culture, social structure, food habits etc. They are distributed in the areas like Dibrugarh, Sibsagar, Dhemaji, Lakhimpur, Jorhat, Sunitpur districts of Assam.

Results

Children's are highly valued by the people of the village Bongalmari. Most of the women bear a child every two or three years during the whole reproductive phase. They also use a contraceptive. Now-a-day they are more conscious about family planning. Some of the respondent's answering my question said that they came to know about their pregnancy when menstruation course stopped for the first time. And they generally went to the Dhemaji Medical Hospital for the confirmation of pregnancy.

The pregnant ladies also performed some of the taboos during pregnancy and this is advised by their mother-in-laws and sister-in-laws. One of the ladies was advised not to kill any animals and not to misbehave with any elderly person. She was also not allowed to go to the burial ground and any ritual integral to death because the evil spirits may harm her embryo. Her husband was also not allowed to kill any animal during that period. Her first two issues were born at home, but the third one is delivered at the Dhemaji Medical Hospital. Some of them are asked to deliver their third issue in the home. It is also mentioned here that generally, they prefer to give birth in the home.

A pregnant lady said that during the birth of her first issue she felt acute pain in the lower part of the stomach. She was taken to her bedroom which was made a female arena. The labour pain was severe, but she was not able to deliver the baby. Then a bamboo mat was placed on the floor of the room which was covered by a cotton sheet. Then she was taken to the mat then she set there in kneel down position. An elderly lady set in front of her and she placed her hands in both of the shoulders of that lady and the expecting lady exerts pressure placing her hands on the tied with *age* (the lower garment of Mishing women) making it just like a rope. After a while, she gave birth a son.The umbilical cord was cut by the other lady with a sharp bamboo split. After birth is gathered in a bamboo basket placing a plantain leaf and attendant woman carried it to the kitchen garden and burned the afterbirth in the kitchen garden by making a hole of about three feet deep.

The newborn was bathed in tepid water and a few drops of honey were given at his tongue. Then the newborn was wrapped with an old and clean cotton cloth and placed by the side of the mother. Some of expecting fathers also promised to god and goddesses during pregnancy that after safe delivery of his wife he will sacrifice two chickens in the deity's name. On the day of purification of mother and child, he scarifies one cock at his residence and the other cock at nearby jungle.

After five days of the birth of the child, a purificatory ceremony is observed known as *aboa:oyolen*, some of the rituals are observed on that occasion and various curries are cooked for the mother made of *malkathi (Splianthes acmela)*, pepper, papaya, *biholongoni (Ptridiun aquilinum),* and chicken. The name giving ceremony of the child is also observed in the first month, and solid food is given to the male child after six to seven months and the girl child after seven-nine months of birth. This ceremony is done by the maternal uncle and the feast is known as *apin sutgod.*

After the birth of the child, the child is introduced to breastfeeding. Time schedule for breastfeeding is not regular; every baby is fed breast milk when it is necessary. Generally, breast milk is fed for two to three years of age of a child. Papaya is eaten by the mother for good production of breast milk.

A good number of postnatal taboos can be observed in the Mishing society integral to childbirth of Bongalmari. Regarding postnatal taboos, my informant said that after the birth of the child she has to face a lot of prohibitions told by her neighbouring elderly women. As the respondent told that she gave birth to a premature child, after the purificatory ceremony the women of the village gathered to tell her about the restrictions. After the ceremony, she could have rice but she was not allowed to eat food before the purificatory ceremony. Milk, tea cannot be taken for a month, she was not allowed to eat green vegetables for one month that the Mishings belief that it causes diarrhea to the child, she is not allowed to eat sour things (*Tenga)* and homemade alkali (*Khar*). Among the fish, she was allowed to eat only small sized fishes and not the big sized one. She was told not to go outside without a knife. She was again not allowed to go to the bank of the rivers and *beels*. She also made her child wear a *najar mala* to save them from the evil eyes. So she performed a lot of taboos during the postnatal period.

We studied the child aged till nine months, so I studied only the cradled baby, answering my question she told that after the birth of the baby her mother-in-law gave a *dola* made with some old clothes like a bed for the newborn. The baby slept at the *dola* for a couple of weeks and then her husband made a cradle for the baby and the cradle was made of bamboo and wood. So, after leaving the *dola* the baby slept in his cradle till nine months age.

Immediate newborn care including cleaning and bathing of the baby is very crucial and thus the newborn should be handled with great gentleness and care. Many infections and a chance of life expectancy are reduced to a large extent through this process. The newborn may even die if the baby is deprived of proper care and favourable environment. Information regarding bath was collected from various women having a child. They said that at their first issue at first they clean the baby with cotton and gave a daily bath to the baby and massage with mustard oil twice a day morning and evening. She used market products for the baby like soap, powder, shampoo, and oil. So, regarding cleanliness, they gave good care to their child.

Toilet training is a very important aspect in child development. It refers to do the habit that the children have to develop to control his bladder as well as the bowel. There is a special time period to start toilet training. It usually occurs as soon as the child attains maturity. A research shows that harsh and punitive measures used for toilet training lead to detrimental consequences on children's personality. The informants said that she taught her two children how to control bladder pressure and latrine and in a day, she also taught them from childhood that how to clean the hands and feet after latrine.

Clothing of the baby is one of the most important measures on child rearing practices. The cloth for the baby should be soft and clean. A respondent answering my question said that she always wrap her child with some soft cotton clothes, she used to clean her baby's cloth so that no infection takes place. Her baby's bed is also covered by soft, clean cotton bed cover, during winter she uses woollen clothes for her baby, she usually uses cotton cloth for the baby, because the cloth is so soft that keeps cool the baby for a longer time, and cotton clothes keep baby cool.

Sleeping is also one of the most important parts of baby's growth. A neonate should sleep for 15-16 hours. To make the baby sleep each and every mother used to sing songs which are known as lullabies. These lullabies are generally not found in written form but have been coming from generation to generation by means of oral tradition. These are generally culture-specific and give many insights into a particular community. Nursery rhymes are usually recited by the adults for children and are also taught at home and schools. Lullabies, nursery rhymes, songs, stories are very fruitful activities through which the young ones are taught words and languages and thus helpful for socialisation. My respondent was a grandmother who used to say that her grandson (aged six months) slept well in the whole day, sometimes he slept for one and two hours in one day, other times he always played. She always made her grandson slept by singing some nice lullabies.

For example:

'"kowwoa kappay pukkaua do: ma: da:,
doduda kablanka dowai,
nollukku kowwomo so kobe patnou,
alagam logbipao douai,
kawbowkou ba bodawo aaptal
gycanae, siminaum bomyoku douai,

tata bongyda sirak aabtoika,
kaubowmou dobpou douai".

(Meaning: O my dear sweet don't cry yourself, when dove will fly, then you cry, who beat my dear child, I shall also beat them, Sweet's father is going for hunting in the jungle, he will catch dear, grandfather will bring pork, sweet will eat rice with those meats.)

The term weaning refers the process by which the baby is changed from its milky diet to other mixed solid diet. After the sixth month of the baby mother's milk cannot give complete nourishment, as the baby grows rapidly at this stage and it needs proper nourishment to attain its maximum growth. Thus, it becomes necessary to introduce other complementary foods in addition to mother's milk. Weaning can be separated into two primary usages. The first sense of the term denotes to the process in which the child is gradually removed from the breast and dependence on breast milk. The second sense of the term refers to the process of introducing semi-solid foods into the infant's diet. In other words, weaning may be partial or complete. In partial weaning the baby is introduced to other foods in the form of liquid, semi-liquid or solid foods, complete weaning is considered to begin only when the baby is totally detached from mother's breast. The process of weaning may have some physiological and psychological consequences. According to some psychological weaning causes great frustration and sudden weaning is traumatic for the child.

Teeth generally come from the month of 6 -7. After eruption of teeth the diet of the child is changed from liquid to solid food items some of the respondents said that the primary solid diets are boiled pulses, boiled rice and fruits mostly banana which is available in that area.

The child starts talking from 10-11 months of age. Different medical facilities like T.T. Vaccination, iron and folic acid etc are given to the pregnant women by the government hospital, again vitamin A, B, C; Hepatitis A, B; polio drops, etc are given to the child.

Health is the most important aspect for children. Although healthcare is equally important at any stage of life, yet childhood period needs more attention than others because of its tender resistance power. The health status of children, proper physical and moral development and general well-being are very much dependent on healthcare practices. In spite of the rapid improvement of medical sciences with sophisticated machines and equipment, modern techniques and drugs, the health status of children in India is still very poor. Many of this mortality and morbidity can be prevented by little awareness and efforts. Such preventive measures are safe drinking water, personal as well as environmental cleanliness and utilisation of available health services.

Common cold: Warm water with salt used for a footbath. After footbath, the child's feet, soles, back, and chest are massaged with warm mustard oil with fried garlic pods.

Fever: The child is wrapped with warm cloth and wet piece folded cloth is kept on the forehead.

Stomach ache, diarrhea: Some herbs such as Indian pennywort (*Centella asiatica*), *masandari* (*Houttujnia cordata*), *mati kaduri* (*Altananthus sessilis*), *pengeri-lata* and curry leaves are reported to have given to the child suffering from diarrhea. For stomach ache mashed *bhim kol* (Musa sp. Colla) is applied on the belly.

A cough: Honey is the common home remedy for treating cough. It was also reported by some mothers of using the juice of basil leaf (black variety) with a few drops of honey.

Cut: Leaves of marrying gold, basil leaves, and raw turmeric are crushed and made a fine paste and tied in the area.

Skin rash, infection, boil, etc.: They generally give a bath to their children with water boiled with *neem* (*Azadirachta officinarum)* leaves. A paste of Indian pennywort applied on boils.

Warm infestation: They generally used bitter things, such as juice of *neem (Azadirachta officinarum), chirata* (wormwood), *and silikha (Terminalia chebula)*.

Injury: Tying paste of raw turmeric in the affected area is reported.

Measles: They generally give a bath to their child with *neem (Azadirachta officinarum)* and basil water.

Asthma: Message with warm mustard oil and garlic as in the case of cold, is reported by the respondents of the Mishing community.

Jaundice: Juice of *kordoi* and sugar cane are given to the children.

Tonsillitis: Sour fruits, cold foods, and water are restricted for the child. The neck portion is covered with cloth so that it would not get a chance to come into contact with a cold breeze.

Constipation: Generally, curry of papaya or ripe papaya is given; warm milk is also given to the baby.

Burn: Mother's milk and saliva are applied in the burnt area.

Nausea and vomiting: Gingers and lime are generally given to get rid of nausea and vomiting.

It is apparent from the present study that the Mishings are very much concern about their children and take care of them with both traditional and modern ways of taking consideration of all the aspects of health of the neonates from the period of pregnancy to the birth of the child and also the infants. They perform all the duties regarding child care in their traditional manner and which help them to keep their traditional knowledge system of child rearing and caring for generation after generation.

References

Baruah, I and P. Bora, 1999. 'Child care and motherhood: A case study among the Sonowal Kacharis of Assam', *Man in India*, 79, 3: 331-345.

Baruah, PC. 2010. *Cultural Traditions and Customary Laws of the Mishings of Assam,* Guwahati; Spectrum Publications.

Bhuiyan, B., 1993. *Child Rearing Practices and Development Status of Children in some Tribal Communities of Assam*, An unpublished thesis submitted to the Gauhati University for the award of Ph.D. degree in Anthropology, Gauhati University, Assam.

Dastidhar, MG and R. Gupta, 1996. 'Infant mortalities and desire for additional children', *Journal of Indian Anthropological Society*, 31:63-69.

Kuppuswami, B., 1980. *A Textbook of Child Development,* Sahibabad; Vikas Publishing House.

Mead, M., 1963. *Coming of Age in Samoa*, New York; Penguin Books.

Muthal, SN. 1992. 'Attitude towards fertility control', *Man in India*, 72, 1: 97-103.

NIPCCS, 1998. *Child Rearing Practices in North Eastern Region- A Study Report*, Guwahati; National Institute of Public Cooperation and Child Development.

Panda, K., 1990. *Elements of Child Development*, p. 93, New Delhi; Kalyani Publishing House.

Rajani, JK.; AVS. Jayalakshmi and TV. Rao, 1979. 'Sex ratios and family welfare programme', *Man in India*, 59, 4: 317-319.

Sharma, KKN and AS. Khan, 1990. 'Fertility and mortality trends of the Khariwar tribal women of Madhya Pradesh', *Man in India*, 70, 4: 446-453.

Sinha, A and H. Pandey, 2000. 'Weaning practices of mothers in Bihar', *Indian Journal of Nutrition and Dietetics*, 37, 10: 338-339.

Srivastava, SL., 1971. 'Birth rites: A comparative study', *Eastern Anthropologist*, 24, 2: 181-195.

Tribhuwan, R and DR. Gambhir, 2001. 'Rural care: The tribal practice of medicine', *Herald of Health,* April, pp. 4-7.

Chapter - 12

A Study of Awareness Concerning Reproductive Healthcare Practices: Experience from the Dibongiya Deoris of Assam

—Juri Borah and Sarthak Sengupta

Introduction

Studies on health status in general and reproductive health, in particular, are an important assignment for enhancing the health awareness among people which in turn help in the socio-economic development of the society. Reproductive health is the most sensitive and imperative part of general health condition. So, a study on reproductive health has to be got notable attention among the people also. The health condition of the people belonging to reproductive age group is associated with the influence of many background characteristics such as education, economic condition, age at marriage, etc. For sound reproductive health each of the partners is equally responsible either biologically or socio-culturally which in turn accountable for their children also. Woman's age at marriage regulates the reproductive span of that particular woman. Lower the age at marriage higher the reproductive span, on the other hand, higher the age at marriage lower the reproductive span. Likewise, mother's age at marriage is closely related to the age of first child birth also. Studies reveal that very low age at marriage or relatively higher age at marriage turns out to be a biologically worrying phenomenon. It is also reported that maternal education is also equally responsible for all of the maintenance of biological condition that has to be faced by an individual. Educated women will get more exposure to have an overall idea or also to perceive the scenario with regards to a reproductive health condition.

Few recent notable works on the level of awareness among different population groups of North East India have been reported by various scholars. Among them Meitei *et al.* (2005: 132-145) worked on the awareness and prevalence of Reproductive Tract Infections (RTI) among the north-eastern states of India in district level. Similarly, Krishnakumari and Arun (2010: 121-130) worked on the reproductive health of women in Andro, Manipur.

Gogoi and Prusty (2013: 8-14) tries to examine the prevalence of reproductive health complications among tribal women and their treatment seeking behaviour in north-eastern region of India based on DLHS-3 data.

Studies on reproductive health problems among rural adolescent girls of Mohanpur block of West Tripura district was done by Baidya *et al.* (2014: 78-82). Shahani (2014: 1-5) also tried to explore the existing practices on sexual and reproductive behaviour among adolescent girls of Meitei-Pangals of Manipur. Again, Deka *et al.* (2015: 51-55) studied the reproductive health and health seeking behaviour of adolescent girls residing in urban slums of Guwahati city.

All these works conducted so far reported about the lack of awareness among the adolescent girls and the women towards their own health condition and consequently have poor reproductive health.

In the present chapter, an attempt has been made to focus on the awareness level concerning various reproductive health issues among the Dibongiya Deori women of Assam.

Materials and Methods

Data pertaining to the present study was collected both from primary as well as secondary sources. The basic information is based on the data collected from 265 ever married women who have at least a live born child from the two exclusively Dibongiya Deori inhabited villages namely, Borchapori and Kinapather Deori besides different Dibongiya Deori settlements at Bihpuria, Bandardewa, and Narayanpur of Lakhimpur district, Assam. A specially designed pretested schedule was used to get relevant data. The information used in this study was gathered during 2014–2016.

The Deori are an indigenous plains Scheduled Tribe of Assam and Dibongiya is one of the major *Khel* (sub-tribe or territorial group) of Deori community, others being Tengaponiya, Borgonya, and Patargonia. It has been reported (Saikia, 1976) that the Patargonia section has become extinct and their existence cannot be traced in any part of Assam. The Dibongiya are the only preserver of their traditional Deori dialect. They belong to a Tibeto-Mongoloid tribal group and mainly concentrated in Lakhimpur, Dhemaji, Jorhat, Majuli, Golaghat, Sibsagar, Dibrugarh and Tinsukia districts of upper Assam and also in the Lohit district of Arunachal Pradesh.

Results and Discussion

The occurrences of various gynecological and obstetric related problems are highly responsible for the poor reproductive health condition of the women. The present study tries to record various gynecological problems experienced by the Dibongiya Deori women. The commonest problem experienced by the present studied Dibongiya Deori women are leucorrhea (No= 63; 23.77 per cent) associated with burning sensation, itching, discomfort, tiredness, etc. Again, 48.30 per cent (No=128) of them have been suffering from menstrual related problems like heavy bleeding, very low bleeding, very low and very high duration of the menstrual cycle as well as irregular bleeding and severe lower abdominal pain during periods. Although modern medical science can resolve such problem within a very short period, the present studied population recorded patients who are suffering from such ailments since last 10 years or more. In this regard, only a few of them are taking regular medicine from doctors while the majority of them totally ignore this issue and consider it as a normal regular phenomenon. Few of them are also taking traditional medicine that is given by traditional healer *(Kichu Liya Mochi)* of the village prepared from various locally available plants. During the investigation, 14.72 per cent of women informed us that they don't consider such type of issue to discuss openly. They believe that if they discuss, it may affect them like a contagious disease. They also mentioned that even they don't want to use the same bank (*ghat*) of the river for washing their clothes having the fear of transmission. Dibongiya Deori women suffering from white discharge are advised by their traditional healer to take medicinal preparations from the root of *satmul* (Garden asparagus, *Asparagus recemosus*) and the paste is mixed with milk and is taken in empty stomach for three consecutive days. When a woman or a girl is suffering from menstruation related problem like lower abdominal pain they take the paste of the leaf of *laijabori* (heart leaf drymary, *Drymaria cordata*) boils it along with garlic and salt and it is taken in empty stomach. It has been observed that even if a woman had experienced occasional bleeding during the caring period they took the help of some traditional folk medicine like using garland (*mala*) prescribed and prepared by the traditional healer of the village. The women who opted for treatment from traditional healers never seek any help from the medical institution even if they fail to get desired results.

Apart from these problems, in response to other gynecological and obstetric problem also they basically prefer traditional medicine.

Reproductive tract infections are the major problems responsible behind unhealthy reproductive health and that are transmittable because of non maintenance of healthy perineal hygiene practices. Proper knowledge and awareness about hygienic practices in this regard are of utmost importance. The present study also enquires about the uses of proper sanitary napkins during the time of menstruation. It is found that women without using any kind of sanitary napkins during menstruation are considerably high (25.28 per cent) among them. Only 23.40 per cent of women use contemporary disposable sanitary napkins while 41.89 per cent of women use old linen or any piece of clothes and about 9.43 per cent of women use both clothes and disposable materials as and when required. The fact stated above may be mainly because of low educational attainment coupled with the poor economic condition. They re-use the same lien piece by washing. Among the users of any kind of napkins, 31.66 per cent of the women use the same napkin for the whole day and 54.27 per cent have changed it for twice in a day. Only 14.07 per cent of women have changed their napkins for thrice and more times during menstruation period. Krishnakumari and Arun (2012: 121-130) mentioned that the frequency of changing sanitary napkins during menstruation is significantly related to infection. Their works among the Andro women found that the women don't take bath during their menstruation period have more reproductive tract infections than the others who maintain the sanitation. Deka *et al.* (2015: 51-55) worked among the adolescent girls residing in urban slums of Guwahati city. Their study reported that majority of the adolescent girls were using old cloth (91.30 per cent) during their menstrual period and 16.2 per cent of girls have changed their napkins for one to two times per day.

The level of awareness of the Dibongiya Deori women regarding Reproductive Tract Infection, Sexually Transmitted Diseases etc. is relatively poor. Only 11.70 per cent women have the knowledge about the possible reason for transmission of AIDS while only 0.38 per cent has the idea about STD i.e., gonorrhea. Friends and relatives constitute a popular source of information among the population. Newspaper, media, health workers, etc. were also served as the source of information. Regarding the knowledge on HIV, it has been observed that 19.62 per cent of the women hear the word AIDS only and nothing beyond else. 38.87 per cent women believe that the transmission of HIV is possible only among those persons who have multiple sex partners and 0.38 per cent believe the mosquito as the cause that brings AIDS. A few women also think that seating with an HIV patient will also bring this disease. Surprisingly, 29.43 per cent of the women didn't hear about the word also. Utterances of such deadly disease also considered as taboo by many of them.

Regarding the health seeking behaviour, it has been observed that many women (9.43 per cent) belongs to somewhat higher ages did not get any medical assistance during their pregnancy period and also they are not aware regarding these matters. But, now-a-days most of the younger generation mothers are becoming interested regarding the improvement of their health condition and have sought the medical assistance from Primary Health Centre (71.70 per cent) and 2.26 per cent women had treatment from an only private physician. 11.70 per cent of them besides availing medical assistance from the governmental organisation, had treatment and advice from a private physician and 1.13 per cent from a traditional healer and 0.38 per cent from village quack also. Besides these, 1.13 per cent and 1.15 per cent of women took help only from the village Quack and the traditional healer respectively. Again 0.75 per cent of women took help from the govt., private physician as well as traditional sources. 24.53 per cent of women had faced the communication and medical problem during pregnancy time. In some remote areas surface communications is deplorable and for that even they use of hand cart or *thela* (0.38 per cent), bicycle (2.26 per cent), rickshaw (0.75 per cent) and also bamboo bier (0.38 per cent) in an emergency. Recently governmental schemes like communication facility (ambulance service) have been launched and quite a good number of mothers are getting the facility.

Now-a-days, health worker (ASHA) visited their village regularly to provide services to the pregnant mothers. But according to the ASHA workers, many people are not interested with regard to the medicine like iron tablets that has been provided by the government free of cost. Regarding the healthcare delivery also it has been observed that out of total birth recorded (including still birth and live birth) the cases of home delivery is more (52.97 per cent) whereas the frequency of delivery at government hospital is 42.21 per cent and also at the private hospital is few (4.82 per cent). Since the mother did not feel any difficulties they prefer home delivery. Of late government has launched various schemes (*mamoni, majoni aachoni*) which provide a token amount of money, few baby products for the new born child and also some nutritious food for the mothers. As such right now women from the present studied village have been preferred delivery at a government hospital. Interestingly, a few women mentioned that although they had given birth their babies at home they availed such aids from the governmental institution.

Abortion is a complex phenomenon that may also affect a woman's overall health condition. The present study reveals the abortion rate (only spontaneous abortion) as 5.03 per cent. The Annual Health Survey (2010-2012: 259-266) reported that the Deoris of Lakhimpur district records the abortion rate (both voluntary and involuntary) as 1.11 per cent per year per 100 women. In this connection, it may be mentioned that the Annual Health Survey Reports cover the all three sub-tribes of Deori population. But the present study has covered only one territorial group of Deori population. Similarly, infant mortality rate among the present studied population is also high (4.78 per cent). From the NFHS report conducted in 1992-1993, 1998-1999 and 2005-2006, it has been revealed that infant and child mortality is considerably high in North East India, varying widely from state to state. The state of Assam records highest mortality rate in North East India which is higher than the average mortality rate of the country. Sometimes the factors responsible for the death of their infant is also difficult to ascertain since many of them are not taking help of any medical expert or medical treatment during the time of their sufferings. They have also a belief in strong supernatural forces with regards to the death of their new born babies.

Women's belief and practices regarding childbirth is also associated with some infections. The cutting of naval cord with unsterilised material brings infection (Krishnakumari and Arun, 2012: 121-130). In the studied population, it has been found that maximum numbers of women who gave birth at home and helped by elderly village women were using sharp bamboo strips for cutting the naval chord (32.83 per cent). This is also a point of concern since it may also be harmful to the mother and the child. Earlier studies conducted by few scholars namely, Nagda (1992: 179), Rao (2008), Reddy and Bharati (2003: 315-336), Bindu (2005), Giridhar *et al.* (2011: 1-11) etc. reported the use of bamboo strips, kitchen knife, sickle or sharp edge or an arrow, wood or stone, either new or old shaving blades or other sharp instruments for cutting the naval cord.

The dried naval cord of the new born baby is considered as the important and essential item for their better health condition. As such it is preserved in a casket prepared from the cocoon of silkworm (63.40 per cent) and tied with a rope to the newborn baby's hand for that it would protect them against unwanted forces. Before wearing it is dried in the sunshine and concerns to keep it away from the birds that are believed to be brought illness condition. Again, when a baby is suffering from fever or stomach problem the same is kept in a glass of water and that water is given to the patient. 3.40 per cent of the mothers used the naval cord as a locket and put on the baby's neck as a locket in the chain and 15.8 per cent of the mothers kept it just to follow the tradition. But, 17.36 per cent of the women either lost or threw it and didn't give importance on it. In this connection, it may be said that although it is their traditional belief system to use the naval cord for children's better health, maintenance of hygienic condition during preserving is also necessary.

The role of Dibongiya women in domestic chores is more than a male person. The entire domestic tasks like carrying heavy water buckets from a distance, cultivation in paddy field and also in kitchen garden is generally done by females. They even do heavy works until the time of delivery also. But they follow some restrictions that they do not across the rope, open the hand oven towel that was used for caring paddy seed and even refrain from weaving and cutting during carrying stage to avoid complicacy.

The very low gap between two children is considered as problematical for the mother and her child (Bhende and Kanitkar, 2010). Among the Dibongiya Deori women, the gap between two children is also very short; 5.28 per cent and 37.36 per cent of the women gave born their babies within one and two years gap respectively. They have a belief system that if the mother disposed of the after birth materials of the parturition stage to a far distance place, then the mother will not conceive once again quickly. Non-success in this regard was also reported by the respondent women in the studied population. It is reported from the work of Barua (1998) that among the Tai Khamyangs the placenta is buried within the compound and also having a belief that deeper the pit bringing the larger gap between two issues.

Regarding the adoption of family planning method, it has been observed that the frequency of non-users (55.80 per cent) is more than the users. Among the non-users, 0.38 per cent of the woman became separated because of religious factor. About 44.15 per cent of the women were found to be using various contraceptive methods where the younger generation mostly prefers oral contraceptives.

During the time of carrying stage, the Dibongiya mother does not take any special diet. Their prescribed diet is similar to the other members of the family. Sometimes few women prefer various locally available vegetables like *koldil* (banana flower), *Kol Pacala* (banana shoot), *kocu* (taro), *tagodhiya* (sweet potato, *Ipomoea batatas*), etc. from their own vegetable garden. These food items are used to enrich iron to the pregnant mother. Many of them are using the homemade rice beer *(suje)* for stimulation during the time of pregnancy.

Among the Dibongiya Deori, 18.11 per cent of mother breast fed their child up for one year or one and a half year, 46.42 per cent of mothers could feed their infants up to three years and 17.36 per cent of mothers' breast fed the child more than three years. During the period of investigation 48 mothers (18.11 per cent) were at the lactating stage, a period which ranges from a newborn baby to three years. The main reasons for weaning are a lower amount of breast milk (2.64 per cent), immediate pregnancy (34.72 per cent), due to working condition (0.75 per cent), and natural (42.64 per cent) others like teeth problem of the baby (0.38 per cent). The level of knowledge on colostrums was also found to be low. Only 40.48 per cent of the women have the knowledge on colostrums. They have a belief that if a new born child is directly breast feed then the child will face discomfort in the toilet. The first breast milk is soaked in a cloth to avoid its fall into the ground. Otherwise, the mother will suffer from an inadequate production of breast milk, they believe. When the mother suffers from an insufficient amount of milk she is given some locally available herbs like *gakhiroti bon* (asthma weed, *Euphorbia hirta*), *Garia aalu* (sweet potato, *Ipomoea batatas*) etc. On the contrary when the mother has an excess amount of milk she is given *mecaki* (Duggal fiber tree, *Debregeasia wallichiana*) to lessen the amount.

Summary

The Dibongiya Deoris are known for their religious bend of mind. The present study records inadequate knowledge on reproductive health issues among the Dibongiya Deori women. Although many of them accepted the modern healthcare facilities offered by the government, yet a considerable number of mothers have experienced various gynecological and obstetric related health problems for prolonged period without any treatment. Health seeking behaviour needs to be improved by making the healthcare services easily available to the Dibongiya Deori woman and at a lower cost. In addition to the existing healthcare facilities in the area of Dibongiya Deori habitation, the additionally specialised centre may be opened up to provide better quality care. Development of various schemes or programmes regarding health education will be of utmost importance to bring awareness regarding personal hygiene, knowledge of various communicable diseases etc.

Acknowledgement

We are thankful to the women respondent and also the inhabitants of the village Borchapori, Kinapather and also different Dibongiya Deori settlements at Bihpuria, Bandardewa, and Narayanpur of Lakhimpur district, Assam whose active participation, and unhesitating interaction make it possible for smooth conduct of data collection.

References

Baidya, S.; M. Debnath and R. Das. 2014. 'A study of reproductive health problems among rural adolescent girls of Mohanpur block of West Tripura district', *Al Ameen Journal of Medical Science*, 7, 1: 78-82.

Barua, I. 1998. 'Socio-cultural and environmental factors of health and economy: A case study of Tai Khamyangs of Assam'. In MK. Bhasin and SL. Malik (Eds.): *Contemporary Studies in Human Ecology,* Delhi: Indian Society for Human Ecology.

Bhende, AA. and T. Kanitkar. 2010. *Principles of Population Studies* (Twentieth edition). Mumbai: Himalayan Publishing House.

Bindu, S. 2005. 'Social structure, child-rearing practices and behaviour pattern among the tribes of Kerala', *Unpublished Ph.D. Thesis, Department of Anthropology, Pondicherry University.*

Deka, C.; AC. Baishya and J. Ojah. 2015. 'A study of reproductive health and health seeking behaviour of adolescent girls residing in urban slums of Guwahati city', *The New Indian Journal of OBGYN,* 2,1: 51-55.

Giridhar, L.; RS. Rao; G. Lakshmi and KB. Swamy. 2011. 'Umbilical Cord Care Practices among the Newborns of Gadaba and Konda Dora Tribes', *Indian Journal of Maternal and Child Health*, 13, 4: 1-11.

Gogoi, M. and RK. Prusty. 2013. 'Reproductive health complications among tribal women in India: A special focus on North East India', *Etawah Journal of Social Sciences*, 8-14.

Hazarika, P. and N. Chutia, 2013. 'Abortion incidents, still birth and reproductive health risk of Deori and Mishing women in the North East India', *International Journal of Science and Technology Research*, 2, 13: 259-266.

Krishnakumari, P. and MC. Arun. 2010. 'Reproductive health of women in Andro', *Journal of the Anthropological Society of Manipur India*, 1: 121-130.

Meitei, MH.; K. Latashori and Ksh. Gopal. 2005. 'Awareness and prevalence of reproductive tract infections in northeast districts of India', *Health and Population-Perspective and Issues*, 28, 3: 132-145.

Nagda, BL. 1992. *Social Correlates of Fertility*. Udaipur: Himanshu Publications.

Rao, RS. 2008. 'Knowledge, attitude and practices (KAP) regarding RCH care among the tribes of Vizianagaram District- a situational analysis', *A report submitted to Tribal Cultural Research and Training Institute, Hyderabad, (unpublished).*

Reddy, S. and Bharati. 2003. 'Beliefs and practices related to parturition among the Konda Reddis of Andhra Pradesh', *Man in India,* 83, 3&4: 315-336.

Saikia, PC. 1976. *The Dibongias.* New Delhi: B.R. Publishing Corporation.

Shahani, R. 2014. 'Adolescence and reproductive behaviour: A study of Meitei-Pangals of Manipur', *International Journal of Scientific and Research Publications*, 4, 9: 1-5.

Vital Statistics Division. 2012. *Annual Health Survey, Assam – 2011-2012 Fact Sheet.* New Delhi: Office of the Registrar General and Census Commissioner, India.

Chapter - 13

Indigenous Health Practices among the Oraon of Assam

—Bhaskar Das

Introduction

Ethnomedicine is an important area which is studied under medical anthropology and it brings to light the different traditional medicines used by the simpler societies for their healthcare practices. It is a set of empirical practices embedded in the knowledge of a social or ethnic group often transmitted orally from generation to generation with the intent to solve health problems. It is an alternative to western medicine and is strongly linked to religious beliefs and practices of indigenous cultures (Bussmann and Sharon, 2007).

Assam is home to numerous ethnic communities including the tea garden workers which constitute one-fifth of the total population in the State. The tea garden community comprises several castes and tribal groups migrated to Assam from different States in India during the British colonialism. Although the major indigenous populations in Assam are more or less studied with regard to their ethnomedicinal beliefs and practices similar studies among the tea garden workers are scanty. At this backdrop, the present study is carried out among the Oraon of Singlijan Tea Estate in Dibrugarh district with regard to their knowledge and indigenous methods of treatment for diseases.

Originally the Oraon is said to have lived in the Deccan, South India before they migrated to the Chotanagpur plateau especially in the State of Jharkhand. Both racially and linguistically they have a close affinity to many South Indian communities. Their language is called *Kurux* which belongs to the Dravidian group of languages. The Oraon is the single largest ethnic group among the tribes found in the Central Tribal belt and the third largest tribe in India. They are brought to Assam by the Britishers to work as tea garden workers. Among the tea garden, tribal populations in Assam the Oraon has got the highest numerical strength.

Subjects and Methods

The study is carried out among the Oraon of Singlijan Tea Estate which is considered as one of the oldest Tea Estate in the Upper Assam region. It is situated around 20 Km East of Dibrugarh town. The present data is collected in the month of March 2013 after taking prior informed consent from the respondents. Information on medicinal plants and indigenous health practices are collected from the traditional herbal practitioners and persons who carry out exorcism (*hard*). Common villagers are also asked regarding the efficacy of the herbal practitioners and exorcists. Standard anthropological methods like a case study, interview and observation are mainly followed.

Findings

The Oraon settlement in Singlijan has 250–300 households. The ex-tea garden labourers stay in their individual houses while the working class lives in personal as well as in the company owned quarters. Originally they are Hindu (*Sarna*) but now many are found converted to Christianity.

There are two herbal practitioners in the village. The villagers approach them for diseases like jaundice, pneumonia, gastric, diarrhea, dysentery, stomach ache, fever, toothache etc. Other than the indigenous herbal practitioners there are two women who carry out exorcism (*jhara*) for jaundice. It is reported that jaundice is quite common among the Oraon of Singlijan and treatment is mostly done by the indigenous methods which include exorcism. Equally common is the incidence of pneumonia which happens to be one of the reasons for child deaths in the village. While there is no available herbal treatment for pneumonia in children below five years of age but in adults, the indigenous mode of treatment using leaves of key lime, black pepper, bonduc nut and watercress is reported to be quite effective. The methods of treatment for diseases as described by the indigenous herbal practitioners are enumerated below:

Jaundice

The symptoms usually observed by the practitioners in patients with probable jaundice are the yellowish colour of skin, eyes, and urine, very low appetite, vomiting, headache, continuous fever etc. A blackish-brown skin associated with brownish sclera is the other occasional symptom for this disease. There are three types of indigenous treatment available in Singlijan for suspected cases of jaundice.

A handful of five-leaved chaste tree leaves (Local name–*Posotia*; Scientific name–*Vitex negundo*; Family–Verbanaceae) is crushed and mixed with water and kept in a bottle after filtering. For an adult, the dose is ½ cup before food and it is taken twice daily for 2–3 weeks. In children, the dose is adjusted accordingly. With this treatment, the patient usually gets cured within 3–4 days. This medicine is not administered to children below five years of age.

This treatment is a type of exorcism (*jhara*) carried out on the patient for three days which is followed by oral intake of indigenous herbal medicine. It is generally carried out in the morning hours. The patient is made to seat facing towards east. A small bowl with a moderate quantity of mustard oil is taken. It is then kept on the patient's head and the mustard oil is stirred with a bunch of *dhub* or Bermuda grass (Local name–*Duboriban*; Scientific name–*Cynodon dactylon*; Family–Poaceae) for 15–20 minutes. Subsequently, the colour of the oil becomes white which is an indication that the patient has jaundice. The Exorcist neither chants anything while carrying out this activity nor does she think that the disease is the act of an external agent. She simply prays to God before the exorcism. After three days the patient is given an herbal medicine which is a combination of turmeric rhizome (Local name–*Halodhi guti*; Scientific name–*Curcuma longa*; Family–Zingiberaceae), five or seven numbers of myrobalan (Local name–*Hilikha guti;* Scientific name–*Terminalia chebula*; Family–Combretaceae) and small amount of jaggery. The ingredients are grinded and mixed and divided into seven equal doses. The medicine is taken thrice daily with raw milk. It is reported that this herbal treatment is not administered in children below five years of age.

It is also a type of exorcism carried out by a woman in the village to treat jaundice. She is not an herbal practitioner but only an exorcist for jaundice. The patients generally get cured after her exorcism and do not require any indigenous herbal treatment. She does not carry out this exercise in small children who are less than two years of age. They are referred to the health centre. However, from 2 to <10 years, this process is carried out above the navel after making the patient lie down. A cone shaped object is prepared with a thick piece of paper after passing it with a molten candle. A small piece of cloth which should be white in colour is kept on the stomach. The cone is then placed on that white piece of cloth just covering the navel portion with the pointed portion facing upward.

The lower part of the cone is covered in a circular manner with a piece of cloth to enable any air to pass. Subsequently, the pointed part of the cone is lit up and two third of the same is allowed to burn. When the remaining part of the burnt cone is removed it is observed that a small amount of sticky yellowish substance gets accumulated on the piece of white cloth. The yellowish colour indicates that the patient has jaundice. This type of exorcism is normally done for a minimum of five days. Usually, the patient gets relief within 5–9 days depending on the severity of the disease. It may be noted that the exorcist while carrying out her exercise does not chant or spell anything. She also does not believe that the disease is due to some supernatural power. For patient >10 years of age, the mode of treatment is same only that it is carried out on one of the ears. Boiled food is advised during the course of treatment and food prepared with mustard oil, meat, egg, oily fish etc are some of the prohibited food items which the patient should avoid until he/she is fully cured.

Pneumonia

Indications for pneumonia are continuous high fever, cough accumulation in chest resulting in breathing difficulty and chest pain. For treatment, 19 or 21 numbers of key lime leaves (Local name–*Gul nemu*; Scientific name–*Citrus aurantifolia*; Family–Rutaceae), 17 or 19 numbers of black pepper (Local–*Jaluk*; Scientific name–*Piper nigrum*; Family–Piperaceae), three numbers of bonduc nut (Local–*Leta guti*; Scientific name–*Caesalpinia crista*; Family–Caesalpiniaceae) and small amount of watercress (Local–*Bon sariah*; Scientific name–*Nasturtium indicum*; Family–Brassicaceae) are grinded and mixed properly. Eight to nine rounded pellets are made out of it and the adult dose is one pellet three times daily in empty stomach.

Gastric

The Oraon of Singlijan is familiar with two types of herbal treatment for gastric:

Burning sensation in neck or chest occasionally associated with diarrhea and stomach ache are symptoms for suspected case of gastric. For preparation of the herbal medicine a handful of small knotweed roots (Local name–*Chimti hak*; Scientific name–*Polygonum plebeium*; Family–Polygonaceae), 250 gms of garlic (Local name–*Rasun*; Scientific name–*Allium sativum*; Family–Liliaceae) and 9 or 11 numbers of clove (Local name–*Laung*; Scientific name–*Syzygium aromaticum*; Family–Leguminosae) are grinded and mixed. Water is then added to it and the liquid is poured into a 200 ml bottle after filtering. The dose for an adult is 50 ml three times daily before food.

Gastric can also be cured when marble shaped pellet made with five leafed chaste tree leaves are taken orally. The dose is one pellet two or three times daily before food. In minors, the dose is adjusted accordingly.

Diarrhea

A handful of Henna leaves (Local name–*Jetuka;* Scientific name–*Lawsonia inermis*; Family– Lythraceae) and three guava leaves (Local name–*Madhuri aam*; scientific name–*Psidium guajava*; Family–Myrtaceae) are crushed to extract juice. One teaspoonful of the same is prescribed three times daily to the adult patients. In children of five to six years of age, the dose is prescribed accordingly.

Diarrhea associated with stomach ache/blood dysentery/fever/gall bladder problems.

Apart from jaundice and gastric, leaves of five leafed chaste tree are used to cure diarrhea associated with a stomach ache, blood dysentery, fever and gall bladder problems. The mode of treatment reported is same for all the diseases. The marble shaped pellet is prepared with five leafed chaste tree leaves. The dose is one pellet two or three times daily before food which is taken orally. In children above five years or so the dosage is adjusted accordingly. The pellets also act as a blood purifier and to get rid of lethargy.

Dysentery

Juice of wild banana plant (Local name–*Bhim kol*; Scientific name–*Musa balbisiana*; Family–Musaceae) is collected after cutting a portion of it. It is then given orally to patients with dysentery. The adult dose is two teaspoonful three times daily.

Toothache

Roots of lemon scented prickly ash (Local name–*Lata tezmui*; Scientific name–*Xanthoxylum nitidum*; Family–Rutaceae) are crushed and the juice is applied on the affected tooth to get relief from pain.

Conclusion

Exorcism related to jaundice is also reported among the Khamyang of Assam (Sonowal and Barua, 2011). Five-leaved chaste trees, an important medicinal plant among the Oraon of Singlijan is found to be used even by the Khamyang for a disease like eczema (Sonowal and Barua, 2011) and Mishing of Upper Assam for pain, body ache and stress (Das, 2014). Small knotweed as elaborated in the present chapter for the preparation of herbal medicine for gastric is reported to be consumed as a leafy vegetable by the Oraon of Jharkhand as it got medicinal properties to cure a cough, dysentery, lactation and gastric (Kumari and Kumar, 2001).

Although the indigenous methods of treatment found among the Oraon of Assam has many limitations but the traditional knowledge recorded is worth preserving. Further, the methods and techniques of treatment used by them need to be scientifically tested for a much wider practice.

References

Bussmann, RW and D. Sharon, 2007. *Plants of Longevity: The Medicinal Flora of Vilcabamba*. Trujillo, Peru (Los Autores).

Das, B. 2014. 'Ethno-medicinal practices among the Mishing: A case study'. In K. Jose and GK. Bera (Eds): *Indigenous Resource Management in North East India*. pp. 152-157, New Delhi; Omsons Publications.

Kumari, B and S. Kumar, 2001. 'A checklist of some leafy vegetables used by tribals in and around Ranchi, Jharkhand'. *Zoos' Print Journal* 16, 3: 442-444.

Sonowal, R and I. Barua. 2011. 'Ethnomedical practices among the Tai-Khamyangs of Assam, India'. *Ethno Medicine*. 5, 1:41-50.

Chapter - 14

Traditional Healing Practices of Forest Fringe Dwellers: A Paradigm of Cost-Effective Medication

—*Samrat Sengupta and Anindita Deka*

Introduction

The traditional system of medicine based on folklore has been in practice since time immemorial, dating back to the beginning of civilisation and this knowledge has evolved over generations of experience, necessity, and practice (Lalramnghinglova, 2000). Traditional healing practices fall under the study domain of "ethnomedicine", which according to Foster and Anderson (1978), denotes the "totality of health knowledge, values, beliefs, skills, and practices of indigenous people, including all the clinical and non-clinical activities that relate to their health needs". Hughes (1968) refers ethnomedicine as "those beliefs and practices relating to disease which are the products of indigenous cultural development and is not explicitly derived from the conceptual framework of modern medicine".

Over the past decade, traditional healing practices using natural herbs have become a topic of global significance in all corners of the world. According to WHO, 80 per cent of the rural population in developing countries utilise locally available medicinal plants for their primary healthcare needs (Pareek, 1996; Syiem, 1999) accounting about not less than 20,000 species of flowering plants being used as medicinal plants (Gupta and Chadha, 1995).

Medicinal plants play an important role in supporting primary healthcare system in India with the practice of ethnomedicine or folklore medicine playing pivotal role among the tribals and non-tribals for the treatment of various diseases and ailments. India is one of the twelve mega biodiversity centres having about 10 per cent of the world's biodiversity wealth. Out of 17,000 species of flowering plants reported to occur in our country, 7500 are known to have medicinal uses and used in traditional and folklore remedies (Sajem and Gosai, 2006). Moreover, there are about 53 million tribal people belonging to 550 communities of 227 ethnic groups and they inhabit about 5000 forest villages (Prakash *et al.,* 2008), representing one of the greatest emporia of ethnobotanical wealth (Chowdhuri, 2000). Ayurveda, the oldest medical system in the Indian Subcontinent, has alone reported approximately 2000 medicinal plant species, followed by the Siddha and Unani medical system (Kala and Sajwan, 2007). Despite the richness of indigenous knowledge among tribal communities and governance systems of sustaining local biodiversity through informal institutions, such invaluable wisdom and heritage are often not documented or given due priority thereby presenting a big research lacunae. Keeping this in mind, Jain (1981) made an extensive review of ethnobotanical studies in India and emphasised works in North-eastern part of India.

North-eastern India situated along the Himalayan region, encompassing major zoogeographic realms - the Indian, the Indo-Malayan and the Indo-Chinese (Olson and Dinerstein, 2002) as well as being the meeting point of the Himalayan region with the Peninsular India (Takhtajan, 1988) harbours about 50 per cent of the total flora of India (around 10,000 species; Chauhan, 1983). Equally diverse are the people who have co-existed with these resources forming an intricate bond. Comprising of eight states, with more than 130 major tribal communities of the total 427 tribal communities found in India (Sengupta, 2013), this region represents an ethnic tapestry of many hues and shades. Due to its strategic location and rugged topography, its inhabitants have scattered and far-flung settlements in remote areas with adjoining forest without modern facilities which have compelled them to depend upon the rich floral diversity for their primary healthcare (being easily accessible and affordable) and by doing so generation after generation they preserve this rich lore of medicinal plants through oral tradition (Yinegar and Yewhalaw, 2007). So far the different authors from North East region have reported 1953 ethnomedicinal uses from this region alone (Dutta and Dutta, 2005).

Of the eight states, Assam comprises 12.8 per cent of the total tribal population of India with 14 hill tribes; 12 of these are tribes whose settlements go back to the days of undivided Assam. The folk culture is still vital in this region. For its richness of plant wealth and diversity of vegetation, Assam is often referred to as the Floristic Gateway of India (Takhtajan, 1988). The occurrence of a number of endemic plant species and most primitive angiosperms has also been reported from some interior parts of the State. Moreover, it is rich in medicinal plant species. A good number of research works have been contributed on medicinal plants during the last two decades from this region (Bhattacharjee *et al.,* 1980; Bora, 1999; Borthakur, 1981, 1997; Borthakur and Goswami, 1995; Gogoi and Boissya, 1984; Tiwari *et al.,* 1979), reporting so far about 350 species having medicinal values. Yet exhaustive studies on ethnomedicinal aspects covering remote forest fringe dwellers of the state have hardly been conducted. Though some of the tribal medicines have already been incorporated in the organised systems of medicine, much larger number of folk medicines has remained endemic to certain pockets or too small geographic regions or to ethnic groups, thus making the area a prospective field for ethnomedical study. However, this time-tested traditional knowledge is now on the verge of extinction for most of the practices are no more in vogue.

From the very ancient time, the traditional system of medicines has been followed from one generation to another verbally among the rural and tribal people and there are no written records of traditional uses of several herbal medicinal plants. Due to remoteness, inaccessibility and closed culture tradition, vast body of ethnobotanical knowledge have remained largely unexplored. Moreover many conservation areas rich in biodiversity are characterised by cultural diversity, but the people who inhabit these areas are often marginalised (Anonymous, 1994, 1996). Moreover, there is a steady decline in human expertise capable of recognising medicinal plants due to modernisation. Political and socioeconomic changes, modern education, the advent of a new style of living, vocations and cultural invasion jeopardize this delicate bond threatening the survival of the genetic resources amounting to a great loss of natural heritage (Chauhan, 1983). If the rich traditional knowledge base of the various ethnic tribes is not documented, then there may come a time when this valuable information which forms the basis of modern medicine, may be lost forever. Therefore, it is becoming an urgent need to record traditional system of medicine, their germplasm collection, cultivation and preservation in a sustainable way. There is also a need for the development of a common platform for traditional healers and their methodology of use to be modified for longer use of prepared medicines. This is to initiate their proper scientific management and exploitation for the economic development of the area.

In the present work an attempt has been made to determine and inventories the status of medicinal plants and their uses by the local community people settled in the fringe villages of Hollongapar Gibbon Sanctuary (hereafter HGS) Jorhat, Assam. HGS is one fine example where both natural processes and human management systems have generated and sustained a vast array of genetic, species and ecological diversity. The people living in the fringe areas of HGS have been residing here since ages and thus have evolved their culture and tradition, myths and folktales in close association with nature and have an intricate relationship/ understanding of the forests and natural resources. A rich diversity of both of population and flora in this region has provided an initial advantage to its inhabitants for observing, and scrutinizing the rich flora of the sanctuary for developing their own traditional knowledge. With the passage of time, they have developed a great deal of knowledge on the use of plants and plant products in curing various ailments, developing a deep-rooted belief in their native folklore medicine for remedies and they rely exclusively on their own herbal cure.

Material and Methods

The study was conducted with an aim to explore highly economic medicinal wealth along with a traditional method of treatment by the local community people settled in the fringe villages of HGS (Jorhat, Assam). HGS (N 26°40'- N 26°45', E 94°20'- E 94°23') is located on the south bank of the mighty Brahmaputra River in the far North East of India (Figure 14.1). For this, extensive field surveys were made (by S. S) from September 2015 to March 2016. To collect information on the medicinal uses of plants several visits to the fringe villages within the study area was carried out. Information on ethnomedicinal plants was gathered from the village chiefs (*gaonburah*), and the traditional healers (*bej/kabiraaj*) applying different tools of participatory approaches such as informal interview, Participatory Rural Appraisal, Key Informant's Interview and Focus Group discussion. Moreover, detailed household surveys using a semi-structured questionnaire with open-ended questions were conducted in the fringe villages to gather information about the trend and prevalence of use of medicinal herbs locally and correlated with demographic pressure and their socio-economic status. This survey was the main source of quantitative information about the traditional healing practices used by the fringe villagers. For trend study, knowledge of each informant was gauged in terms of the number of ethno-species reported by him. The highest number of ethno-species reported was taken as 100 per cent and percentage of each number reported by each informant was then calculated. It was assumed that greater the number of species reported by the informant more was his ethnomedical knowledge. The herbalists consulted were convinced about the importance of documentation of ethnic knowledge about the medicinal plants used for various curative purposes. Prior informed consent of the village chiefs and other respondents were obtained before conducting the interview and questionnaire survey and also a prior informed consent (PIC) was obtained from the community to share and publish the facts relating to the traditional healing practices used by them. Our study draws heavily on secondary information, thus tactful handling and persuasion to bring out the authentic information from the herbal practitioners were given prime importance.

All the plant's specimens reported to be in use for traditional healing practices were collected in its flowering stage for identification. Incomplete specimens (as for example, only bark material) were also collected and recorded for future collection and documentation. Routine methods of plant collection and herbarium technique have been followed in the study (Jain and Rao, 1977; Alexiades, 1996). All relevant information about the plants were recorded with regards to their vernacular names; plant parts used, the process of preparation of medicine, either individually or in combination with other plant parts, and mode of application both during personal interviews and questionnaire surveys. The doses for the treatment of a particular disease or diseases were also recorded. These specimens were identified using relevant floras and standard literature (Hooker, 1989); Kanjilal *et al.*, 1982). Voucher specimens have been submitted to the

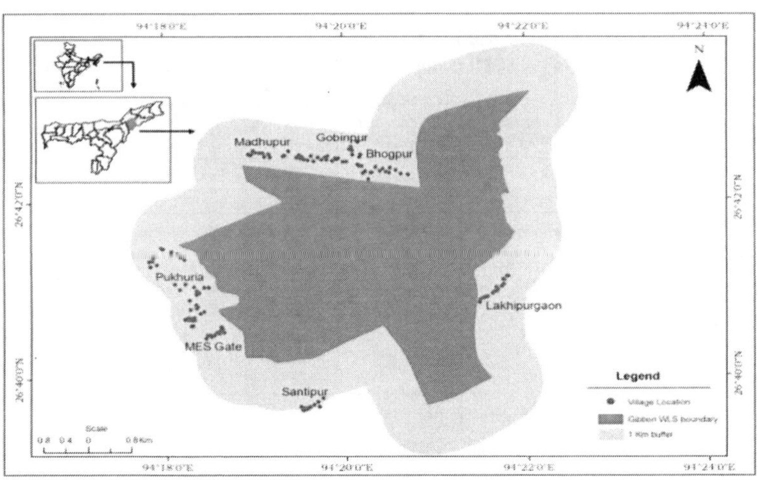

Fig. 14.1: Map showing study area and sampled household location in the Fringe villages of Hollongapar Gibbon Sanctuary, Jorhat, Assam.

Department of Ecology and Environmental Science, Assam University, Silchar and confirmation of identification was done by consulting the taxonomist from Botanical Survey of India, Shillong.

The plants were described in Table 14.1 according to alphabetic order of botanical name. The vernacular (local) name (s) and the name of the families have also been provided along with the valid botanical name. From a total of seven villages, comprising a total of 1055 households (3062 villagers; 1524 men and 1538 women) in the study area, ≥ 10 per cent households (n=161) were selected by simple random sample technique for the household level survey.

Results and Discussion

In Table 14.1, we have enumerated 97 plants alphabetically, giving information on the botanical name and synonym (if any), family and vernacular name that has been traditionally used for treating the ailments by the village elders as well as traditional healers for different major ailments. This is followed by details of parts used, disease type, a method of preparation and dosages and any other uses if present if details provided with. A cumulative list, where different villages reported different uses of medicinal herbs along with ethnicity, demographic profile of each village has also been provided (Table 14.2). On systematic positioning of the plants used in the system of treatment, it was found that distribution of plant was common in the families of Lamiaceae (5), Asteraceae (4), Lauraceae (4), Moraceae (6) and Zingiberaceae (4).

Table 14. 1: List of Medicinal Plants used by the ethnic communities residing in the Fringe villages of Hollongapar Gibbon Sanctuary, Jorhat, Assam

Sl. No.	*Scientific Name*	*Family*	*Common Name*	*Medicinal Use*
1.	*Achyranthes aspera* L.	*Amaranthaceae*	*Bon-sodh*	Juice of the aerial parts mixed with water taken orally against intestinal worms.
2.	*Ageratum conyzoides* L.	*Asteraceae*	*Gendhali bon*	Leaves are used to prevent bleeding in cuts and wounds
3.	*Allium sativum* L.	*Liliaceae*	*Rasun*	The bulb is taken orally to reduce high blood pressure. A paste of the bulb is mixed with the paste of *A. sepa* is applied externally on the affected area to cure of cat bite.
4.	*Alocasia acuminata* Schott.	*Araceae*	*Bej- kochu*	Young shoot, tender leaf, and caudex are eaten cooked with acidic fruit. The leaves grinding with dried fish are kept in the bamboo shoot. It is used for malaria and blood purification.

(*Cont'd...*)

5.	*Alpinia alughas* (Retz) Rose	*Zingiberaceae*	*Tora*	Rhizome juice is taken twice daily to cure a cough.
6.	*Alpinia galanga* (L.) Wild	*Zingiberaceae*	*Gandhi Tora*	Rhizomes ate fresh or with betel nut. A small portion of petiole or rhizome is added to curries for flavour.
7.	*Alstonia scholaris* (L.) R. Br.	*Apocynaceae*	*Sotiyona*	The latex of leaves applied to cure boils, Decoction of bark taken in cholera and stomach pain. Boils, skin diseases, and ulcers.
8.	*Alternanthera sessions* (L.) R. Br.	*Asteraceae*	*Mati-kaduri*	Plant grind with the leaves of *Hibiscus Rosa-sinensis* and tied with a piece of cloth in bone fracture and wound.
9.	*Amaranthus spinosus* L.	*Amaranthaceae*	*Kata-Khutara*	Root extract is taken orally in chest pain.4-8 teaspoonful of root juice taken twice daily inurinary obstruction associated with pain and burning sensation.
10.	*Artocarpus heterophyllus* Lam.	*Moraceae*	*Kothal*	Latex applied on skin disease, wound, and Scorpion sting.
11.	*Arundo donax* L.	*Poaceae*	*Nol*	The whole plant is used to keep Rice. It is also used treat "bagly" (skin disease).
12.	*Asparagus racemosus* (Willd.)	*Liliaceae*	*Satmul*	Dried leaves are powdered and taken orally to cure stomach disorders.
13.	*Azadirachta indica* A. Juss.	*Meliaceae*	*Moha Neem*	Affected parts are massaged with *neem* oil in rheumatic pain and taken orally for worms, Leaves are boiled in water and used at the time of bath to prevent infection from smallpox and other skin diseases.
14.	*Baccaurea ramiflora* Lour.	*Euphorbiaceae*	*Khusmai*	Young fruit is prescribed to eat in jaundice.
15.	*Bombax ceiba* L.	*Bombacaceae*	*Himolu*	Root is ground and mixed with water & kept overnight. The juice so obtained is taken orally in empty stomach every early morning to cure white discharge.
16.	*Bryophullum pinnatum* (lam). Kurz.	*Crassulaceae*	*Dupor Tenga*	Leaf extract taken with water in the empty stomach in the morning helps in Urinary problems and for the release of kidney stone.
17.	*Calamus rotang* L.	*Arecaceae*	*Bet*	Leaf juice applied in eye problem and de-worming.
18.	*Camellia sinensis* (l). Kurtz.	*Theaceae*	*Cha*	Green leaves are used to reduce high blood pressure.
19.	*Cannabis sativa* L.	*Cannabaceae*	*Bhang*	Leaf useful in fungal infection of the skin.
20.	*Cassia fistula* L.	*Caesalpiniaceae*	*Sonaru*	A decoction of leaf applied locally on leprosy.

(Cont'd...)

21.	*Catharanthus roseusl.* (L) G. Don	*Apocyna-ceae*	*Nayantara*	Leaf juice is given orally in the morning in empty stomach in diabetes.
22.	*Centella asiatica* (L.) Urb.	*Apiaceae*	*Bor-manimuni*	Infusion of leaf taken in dysentery, cholera and stomach ache. Plant ate as raw or after cooking against worms.
23.	*Chromolaena odorata* (L.) King and H. Rob.	*Asteraceae*	*Jarmani bon*	Juice of leaf applied in allergic and skin disease.
24.	*Cinnamomum bejolghata*	*Lauraceae*	*Patihonda*	Leaf is used as anti-diabetic.
25.	*Cinnamomum tamala* Nees.	*Lauraceae*	*Tezpat*	The leaves are useful in gonorrhea, rheumatism, diarrhea, enlargement of spleen and diabetes.
26.	*Cinnamomum zeylanicum* Breyne	*Lauraceae*	*Dalchini*	The branches of the trees are looped and their bark removed; the dried inner bark constitutes the drug, Cinnamon. The drug is used in diarrhoea, vomiting. It is commonly used as a condiment.
27.	*Cissus quadran-gularis* L.	*Vitaceae*	*Harjora Lota*	A paste of stem used as a bandage on the fractured bone. The application replaced with a fresh application on alternate days for a month.
28.	*Citrus aurantifolia* (Chr.) Sw.	*Rutaceae*	*Kaghzi lebu*	Lime juice is applied for sprains of legs and hands.
29.	*Citrus maxima* (Burm.) Merr.	*Rutaceae*	*Rabtenga*	About 100 ml juice of the fruit mixed with about 30g powder of dried tuber of *Cyperus rotundus* and taken once daily for a week in gynaecological disorder.
30.	*Clerodendron viscosum* Vent.	*Verbenaceae*	*Dhapatita*	Decoction of tender shoot and root taken in malaria, leaf juice is taken orally to reduce high blood.
31.	*Cleroden-drum cloebroo-kianum* L.	*Verbenaceae*	*Nefafu*	Leaves are eaten to reduce high blood pressure and cure jaundice.
32.	*Clitoria ternatea* L.	*Fabaceae*	*Aparajeeta*	In Ulcer, dysentery, poisonous insect bite.
33.	*Cocos nucifera* L.	*Arecaceae*	*Narikal*	Tender coconut water and milk extract are taken for stomach ulcer.
34.	*Colocasia esculenta* (L.) Schott	*Araceae*	*Kala-kachu*	Rhizome paste applied in cuts, burns and scorpion sting, Shoot is used to cure jaundice.
35.	*Coriandrum sativum* L.	*Apiaceae*	*Dhania*	Seeds are given in abdominal pain and diarrhoea.
36.	*Costus speciosus*	*Liliaceae/ Castaceae*	*Jomlakhuti*	Rhizome paste is given in jaundice.

(Cont'd...)

	(Koen.ex. Retz.) J.E.Smith			
37.	*Curculigo orchioides* Gaertn.	*Liliaceae*	*Bon-tamuli*	Rhizome extract used externally in gonorrhea.
38.	*Curcuma zedoary* Bergius	*Zingibera-ceae*	*Kalo Ada*	Use for colic, loss of appetite and indi gestion, Cough and cold and diabetic.
39.	*Cynodon dactylon* (L.) Pers.	*Poaceae*	*Dalisa dubori*	A paste of the plant applied locally in gum bleeding. Fresh juice of the plant taken 2-teaspoonfuls twice daily for 3 days in fever.
40.	*Dillenia indica* L.	*Dillenia-ceae*	*Outenga*	A decoction of floral parts used in amoebic dysentery. Fruit paste applied to check bleeding from cuts.
41.	*Dioscorea alata* L.	*Discoreaceae*	*Kath Alu*	Tubers useful in Anaemia.
42.	*Diplazium esculentum* (Retz.) SW	*Athyriaceae*	*Dhekia*	The tender apical leafy portion is used as a vegetable.
43.	*Emblica officinalis* Gaertn.	*Euphor-biaceae*	*Amlokhi*	Juice of leaf and fruit is taken orally against diabetes.
44.	*Ficus beng-balensis* L.	*Moraceae*	*Bor Gass*	Blood purifier, and also used in a kidney stone.
45.	*Ficus glomerata* Roxb	*Moraceae*	*Dimoru*	Milky juice is applied as a thick layer on the pain area. If it is acute and bone is thought to be fractured, the bark is tied on the affected area together with juice for 15-30 days.
46.	*Ficus hispida* Vahl	*Moraceae*	*Dimoru*	Exudates from root taken in diabetes. Curry prepared from leaf and taken in jaundice.
47.	*Ficus racemosus* L.	*Moraceae*	*Dimoru*	Hearing loss, Blood Disease, Headache.
48.	*Ficus religosa* L.	*Moraceae*	*Ahot*	About 15 ml Bark decoction mixed with a pinch of rock salt taken twice daily for 3 days to women after childbirth to relieve pain.
49.	*Garcinia cowa* Roxb.	*Clusiaceae*	*Kuji thekera*	Dried pericarp boiled with pulps of 2 or 3 fruits of *Terminalia chebula*, one or two half-fried fish and rice gruel (about 250 ml.) taken after childbirth to prevent dyspepsia.
50.	*Garcinia pedunculata* Roxb.	*Clusiaceae*	*Thekra*	Dried slices of fruits are soaked in water and the juice is given in blood dysentery

(*Cont'd...*)

51.	*Gmeliana arborea* Roxb.	*Verbena-ceae*	*Gomari*	Pain in head, diarrhoea, stomach pain.
52.	*Hedyotis scandens* Roxb	*Rubiaceae*	*Bon-jaluk*	A decoction of leaf taken orally to cure urinary and kidney disorder and asthma.
53.	*Hibiscus suddarifa* L.	*Malvaceae*	*Tenga Mora*	Leaves are used in dysentery of man and domestic animals.
54.	*Hibiscus rosasinensis* L.	*Malvaceae*	*Jobaphol*	Boiled juice of flowers is mixed with honey and taken for heart problem.
55.	*Houttuyia cordata* Thunb.	*Saurauaceae*	*Mosandri*	Leaf juice is useful in gastroenteritis.
56.	*Hydrocotyle sibthopi-oides* L	*Apiaceae*	*Haru mani-muni*	The whole plant is used in stomachic disorder and carminative and rice beer preparation.
57.	*Lagerstomea speciosa* (L.) Pers.	*Lythraceae*	*Azar*	2-10 ml decoction of bark taken 3-5 times daily in diarrhoea and dysentery. 5 ml decoction of the root taken orally 2-4 times daily in jaundice.
58.	*Lantana camera* L.	*Verbena-ceae*	*Ghoo-phool*	Leaf paste applied in cuts. A decoction of leaves taken orally in tetanus.
59.	*Lawsonia inermis* L.	*Lythraceae*	*Jetuka*	Leaf paste useful in fever, high blood pressure and effective in fungal infection of the skin.
60.	*Leucas indica* (L.) R.Br.ex Vatke	*Lamiaceae*	*Durun*	Leaf juice is used in sinusitis
61.	*Litsea cubeba* Pers.	*Lauraceae*	*Mejankri*	Decoction of fruit taken orally in colic and heart diseases. A paste of stem bark applied in scabies and eczema.
62.	*Mangifera indica* Lin.	*Anacardia-ceae*	*Aam*	Decoction of bark taken in empty stom ach; twice daily before meal till complete relief from dysentery
63.	*Melastoma malabath-ricum* L.	*Melastoma-ceae*	*Futukola*	Juice of leaf taken in diarrhoea and dysentery. Juice of leaf and flower took in leucorrhoea.
64.	*Mentha spicata* L.	*Lamiaceae*	*Pudina*	Leaves are used as a vegetable and for the treatment of fever and bronchitis.
65.	*Mesua ferrea* L.	*Clusiaceae*	*Nahar*	Paste of flowers applied on cuts to stop bleeding; also used in piles.
66.	*Michelia champaka* L.	*Magnolia-ceae*	*Champa-full*	The paste of bark is used in rheumatism. Women use the root juice in a monthly period.
67.	*Mikania micrantha* H.B. & Kunth	*Asteraceae*	*Ripuji-lota*	Leaf paste applied to stop bleeding from cuts.

(*Cont'd...*)

68.	*Mimosa pudica* L.	*Mimosaceae*	*Lajuki lota*	A paste of young shoots applied in cuts and wounds. Root used externally in a toothache.
69.	*Mimusops elengi* L.	*Sapotaceae*	*Bokul*	Ripe fruit locally applied in insect bite.
70.	*Moringa oleifera* Lam.	*Moringaceae*	*Sojina*	Juice of leaves is applied frequently to remove blackhead pimples.
71.	*Murraya koenegii* Spreng	*Rutaceae*	*Narasingha*	Leaf juice used as a tonic, curing many stomach problems.
72.	*Musa balbisiana* (Rety) Rose	*Musaceae*	*Bhim kol*	Highly nutritious and fruit is used as baby food.
73.	*Nyctanthus arbourt-ristis* L.	*Oleaceae*	*Sewali*	Leaves are used in malaria
74.	*Ocimum basilicum* L.	*Lamiaceae*	*Kola Tulsi*	A paste of leaf applied in Acne and pimples. Leaves are used in a cough and chronic fungal infection.
75.	*Ocimum gratissi-mum* L.	*Lamiaceae*	*Ram tulosi*	The leaf juice is used to cure problem of eye.
76.	*Ocimum sanctum*	*Lamiaceae* Linn	*Tulsi*	Paste of fresh leaves rubbed over infected skin.
77.	*Oldenlandia corymbosa* Linn	*Rubiaceae*	*Banjaluk*	The plant is diuretic, stomachic, carminative and used as a liver tonic. It is also used in jaundice.
78.	*Oroxylon indicum* (L.) Vent.	*Bignoniaceae*	*Bhat-ghila*	Infusion of stem bark taken orally in diarrhoea and dysentery.
79.	*Oxalis cornicu-lata* L.	*Oxalidaceae*	*Tengesi*	Plant paste filtered and used as eye drop in eye diseases, powdered root is applied on teeth to cure a toothache.
80.	*Paederia foetida* L.	*Rubiaceae*	*Bhedai lata*	Decoction of leaves and tender shoot mixed with Oxaliscorniculata plant in equal quantities taken 2-teaspoonfuls twice daily till cure in diarrhoea and dysentery.
81.	*Passiflora assamica* L.	*Passiflorace*	*Noltenga*	The juice of the leaves is astringent and is specific for diarrhoea and dysentery.
82.	*Phlogaca-nthus thyrsiflorus* (Hardw.) Mabberley	*Acantha-ceae*	*Tita phul*	8-10 flowers or 20-30 leaves (fresh or dried) boiled in water and a half cup of decoction taken twice daily for 15-20 days to cure malaria. Extract of flower useful in asthma and smallpox.
83.	*Phyllanthus embllca* L.	*Euphorbiaceae*	*Amlakhi*	Fruits are used in diarrhoea and dysentery, bronchitis, hair medicine

(*Cont'd...*)

84.	*Piper betle* L.	*Piperaceae*	*Pan*	Fresh leaf taken with salt to cure abdominal spasm and colic. Leaf juice is used externally to cure cataract.
85.	*Piper nigrum* L.	*Piperaceae*	*Jaluk*	The fruits are consumed in indigestion, Body ache and in the post labour ailment as well as in the bone fractures.
86.	*Polygonum bractiate* L	*Polygonaceae*	*Noltenga*	A decoction of the leaf is given in Dysentery.
87.	*Polygonum chinense* L.	*Polygona-ceae*	*Madhu seleng*	Leaf juice useful in Dysentery and effective in stomach problem.
88.	*Polygonum orientale* L.	*Polygonaceae*	*Bihlongoni*	By spreading whole plant powder on water, fish can be easily caught.
89.	*Psidium guajava* L.	*Guava*	*Myrtaceae*	A Headache, Toothache, Diarrhoea.
90.	*Stereos-permum chelonoides* (L.f) DC	*Bignoniaceae*	*Paroli*	Used in tuberculosis.
91.	*Swertia chirayita* (Roxb. ex. Flem.)	*Gentianaceae*	*Chirata tita*	Juice of leaves or infusion of the dried part given in fever, indigestion, skin disease.
92.	*Syzygium cuminii* (L.) Skeels	*Myrtaceae*	*Jam*	Powder of dried fruit pulp with sugar is given in blood dysentery. Ripe fruit is eaten raw to cure diabetes.
93.	*Tamarindus indica* L	*Caesalpinia-ceae*	*Teteli*	Juice of the fruit is mixed with water and taken orally in hypertension. Same is applied to the head to reduce high blood pressure.
94.	*Terminalia arjuna* (Roxb. ex. DC.) Wt. & Arn.	*Combreta-ceae*	*Arjun Goss*	The bark is immersed in a glass of water for overnight and the extract is taken in diabetes. The bark is boiled and the juice so obtained is mixed with milk and is taken in heart problem.
95.	*Terminalia chebula* Retz.	*Combreta-ceae*	*Hilikha*	A decoction of seed given once daily for 7 days in asthma. Unripe fruit is useful in medicine for diarrhea and dysentery.
96.	*Thunbergia grandiflora* Roxb.	*Thunbergiaceae*	*Nilkantha*	Leaf paste mixed with hen's egg and taken orally in gastric troubles. Watery juice obtained from nodes inter-node part is applied locally on eyes for treating conjunctivitis.
97.	*Zingiber casumnar* Roxb.	*Zingiberaceae*	*Bura ud*	Paste prepared from rhizome with common salt and given once daily in empty stomach for two days during indigestion and gas formation.

A preliminary study on the ethno-medico-botany of the *Zeme* (Naga) tribe of N.C. Hills recorded 33 species (Tamuli and Saikia, 2004), while another subsequent study added to the above record with new usage of eight species of plants (Rout *et al.*, 2010). Das *et al.* (2002) have reported

72 plant species from 42 families, used against some common ailments of the tea tribes settled in the Barak Valley. Our study documented a high total of 97 species which may be due to the rich floral diversity in and around the protected area along with the rich ethnic assemblage culminating into the diverse use of medicinal plants (Table 14.2).

Table 14.2: List of Forest Fringe villages and ethnomedical use of plants reported in Hollongapar Gibbon Sanctuary, Jorhat, Assam

Sl. No.	*Name of Forest Village*	*Total Male (2011)*	*Total Female (2011)*	*Total Population (2011)*	*Ethnic Communities*	*Ethnomedicinal use of plants reported (n)*
1.	Bhogpur	107	90	197	Assamese	63
2.	Lakhipur	72	63	135	Assamese	47
3.	Santipur	72	71	143	Nepali, Assamese, Bihari, Buddhist, Tea Tribes	59
4.	MES Gate	385	335	720	Nepali, Assamese, Tea Tribes	33
5.	Pukhuria	482	593	1075	Nepali, Assamese, Tea Tribes	51
6.	Madhupur	257	251	508	Assamese	61
7.	Gobinpur	149	135	284	Assamese	27

During the course of study, it was observed that different ethnic groups in the area have similar knowledge of medicinal herbs; however, mode of treatment for different ailments differs in its own way. However, one thing common in all, irrespective of ethnicity is most of the residents have their own home gardens rich in fruit trees, vegetable crops, bamboo species etc. The home gardens are in their immediate surroundings, through which they are able to maintain the beneficial plant biodiversity as a source of medicine and shelter.

They all follow a strict mandate of resource extraction emphasising maturity of the plants, height of the plants, colour and other morphological characters while collecting the medicinal plants so as to ensure that medicinal plants resource do not deplete from the natural habitat. While gathering the medicinal plants from their habitat peoples avoid collecting plants those are infected by insects, pests, and any other disease.

Plants affected by sunstroke, hailstorms, high-velocity winds, and fire are also not collected to be used for the preparation of indigenous medicine.

Even though it was evident from our focal interview that leaf and roots are the most important plant parts used for medicinal purposes, different parts of a single species are also used for the cure of different ailments. These are usually prepared with water and the drugs are administered with cow milk, sugar candy, honey, salt etc. For the application of herbal medicine, most of the remedies are made orally and average or maximum three dosages are used for three to four days only. The number of dosages usually depends upon the severity of the diseases and the age of the patients. The local traditional healers strictly prohibit the use of Ayurvedic medicine during the course of herbal remedy and avoid spicy, oily meat and alcohol during the treatment period.

Eight informants (4.9 per cent) out of total number 161 reported less than 10 medicinal plant uses. Remaining 153 informants reported various uses of medicinal plants. A moderate positive correlation was established between a number of medicinal plants species reported and the age of the informant with correlation coefficient 'r'= 0.66 and was found to be significant at 95 per cent level of confidence (Fig.14.1a). However, a mild negative correlation was established between a number of medicinal plants species reported and the education level of the informant with correlation coefficient 'r'= -0.21 (Fig.14.1b). Significance test of the sample estimate was performed by direct reference to correlation coefficient table. Younger people harbour less knowledge about plants and their various uses. This could be attributed to mainly two reasons. The primary reason could be because of less association of younger people with the older ones as a

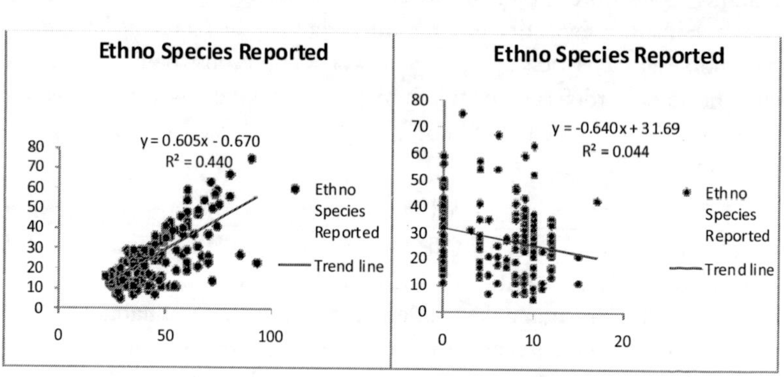

Fig.14.1. Trend of Ethnomedical knowledge of ethnic people (a) along age, and (b) education level around Hollongapar Gibbon Sanctuary, Jorhat, Assam.

result of which the ethnobotanical knowledge could not be transferred to the successive generations efficiently. Secondly, it could be because of the unavailability of desired faunal resources as a result of strict conservation laws of the government.

Choice of herbs depended on several factors, such as the alternatives available, the reputation of a recipe, past experience in the family, access to the plant, and whether it was used singly or in the mixture. These perceptions vary from community to community, and even person to person (Jain, 1991, 1999) which may be a contributing factor in our study. Due to overexploitation and excessive collection of medical plants; researchers keep searching for suitable substitutes to reduce pressure on prime species of medicinal importance. In our study, many species used are co-generic with well known and tested drug species. A few examples are: Anthelmintic: *Clerodendrum colebrookianum* L. is used by the folk, whereas *C. infortunatum* L. is official; for jaundice: *Hedyotis scandens* Roxb. in folk medicine, whereas *H. corymbosa* (L.) Lamk. is official for asthma.

Out of the seven villages studied, five of them are not connected by proper roads and the people have to walk a long distance through non-navigable roads which go through the sanctuary to reach even the nearest town (Mariani). So, traditional medicine has remained as the most affordable and easily accessible source of treatment in the primary healthcare system of resource-poor communities, and the local therapy is the only means of medical treatment for such communities (Yineger and Yewhalaw, 2007).

Conclusion

Ethnobotanical exploration brings out the age-old practices of use of plants to the limelight with possibilities for further exploitation and value addition in the commercial venture as well as for exploitation of new biomolecules for the benefit of mankind. Ethnobotanical studies have led to the documentation of a large number of conventional and non-conventional medicinal plants used by tribals for meeting their multifarious requirements (Dutta and Dutta, 2005).

Tribal people acquired this knowledge of plant species largely on trial and error basis (Pandi *et al.*, 2007) and have entrusted immense faith in their traditional system of medicine which is largely based on traditional cultures, beliefs, and superstition. They have a deep understanding of the ways of nature and the need for the conservation of forest and its product. Almost all the species recorded in the present study were collected from natural habit. Hence there is urgent need to check the overexploitation of natural population and conservation of medicinally potent species of this fragmented forest patch, even when excessive collections and exploitation of medicinal plants are seldom encouraged here. Excessive collections and ruthless exploitation through an unscientific and non-regulated collection of medicinal plants in the recent times by pharmaceutical industries disturbs the regulatory practices, thereby threatening and endangering plants of medicinal value. Plant resources are depleting globally at an alarming rate and at this rate many species of economically and medicinally important plants will become extinct if not controlled. Moreover, a great majority of swallowtail butterflies use medicinal plants for egg laying in the study area (Singh *et al.,* 2015). Loss of medicinal plants due to unplanned extraction and habitat destruction may lead to migration and extinction of many butterfly species.

Socio-cultural attributes have a great bearing in shaping and conserving biological diversity (Pretty, 2003a, 2003b; Singh and Sureja, 2006a, 2006b). Ethnic cultures with ritualistic consideration for plants imbibe veneration for them. Incorporation into biodiversity conservation and ecological studies of local use patterns and of the socio-cultural and institutional background that guides the relationship between people and nature has led to a greater understanding of the relationship between social and biological dynamics (Olsson and Folke, 2001; Gunderson and Holling, 2002). The most important human aspect of biodiversity is the appreciation of the impact of any measures of managing biodiversity on the culture of the people living in close contact with resources. Experience world over is showing that management policies fully involving the indigenous cultures only can be successful on a lasting basis. Biological entities and human societies have to be viewed as codependents. However, Alcorn (1984) emphasised that once a species gets known as a resource in any human society, the impact of this knowledge on expansion, distribution, threats to that species, and in cases even its extinction, play a great role. Thus, this study warrants immediate follow-up detailed ethnobotanical study of its adjoining areas in order to conserve the valuable ethno-medico-botanical knowledge as well as plant resource of this landscape. Unsustainable harvesting from the wild should be stopped and appropriate agro-techniques along with home gardening of some important medicinal plants should be adopted for the effective cultivation of medicinal plants in large scale. Establishment of protected areas, medicinal plant sanctuaries, medicinal/herbal forests, etc is essential for *in situ* conservation of rare herbs. Further, public awareness on ecological niche regime of several medicinal plants could help in a long term conservation perspective. This would not only spread awareness to conserve and preserve the traditional knowledge but also open new avenues to scrutinize these rich natural resources for further studies, development of potential herbal medicines and to the development of the landscape as a whole.

One impending threat that looms large in this landscape is the decline of the practice of herbal medicine among the community people. Some of the major reasons for this are the rapid expansion of small tea growers and increased popularity of allopathic medicines. Moreover, the gradual degradation of natural forests as well as strengthening the regulations by the forest department authority has forced the lifestyle of these people to change in this region. Hence, during last few decades, the choice of the people of this region has taken a distinct turn from actual forest-based livelihood to partial dependence on natural products. To add to the woes, this knowledge is becoming confined chiefly to the folk-healers and old folks residing in villages and is a guarded secret which is handed down by them to any of the son of his choice, or to a daughter if absent. They strictly adhere to the notion that divulging the formulation of a medicine to a patient or others could reduce the effectiveness of the medicine eventually leading to loosening of their professional supremacy.

Our study shows that there is immense potential for ethnobotanical research which would benefit not only the scientific world but also open up new avenues for augmenting the tribal economy through a sustainable approach. The existence and dependence on a large number of traditional practices can be thought of as an alternative type of medicine, where the cost and side effects are negligible. Thus, in the end, we can safely say that traditional healing practices of indigenous people facilitate the development process in cost-effective, participatory and sustainable ways and play an important role in resource conservation. Perhaps after a detailed investigation by modern scientific techniques, at least some of these plants documented here might prove to be effective life-saving drugs plants for cure and relief of various ailments and diseases that plague to mankind.

References

Alcorn, JB. 1984. *Huaestec Mayan Ethnobotany*. Univ. Texas Press, Austin.

Alexiades, MN. 1996. 'Collecting ethnobotanical data: An introduction to basic concept and techniques'. In MN. Alexiades (Ed): *Selected Guidelines for Ethnobotanical Research: A Field Manuel*. pp. 53-94.The New York Botanical Garden, New York.

Anonymous. 1994. *Indigenous Knowledge Systems and Biodiversity Management*. International Centre for Integrated Mountain Development, Kathmandu.

Anonymous. 1996. *Banking on Biodiversity*. International Centre for Integrated Mountain Development, Kathmandu.

Bhattacharjee, S, KC. Tiwari, R. Majumdar and AK Misra,1980. 'Folklore medicine from district Kamrup (Assam)'. *Bulletin of Medico Ethnobotanical Research* 1: 447-460.

Bora, PJ, 1999. 'A study on ethnomedicinal uses of plants among the *Bodo* tribe of Sonitpur district Assam'. *Journal of Economic and Taxonomic Botany* 23: 609-614.

Borthakur, SK,1981. 'Studies in ethnobotany of *Karbis (Mikirs):* Plants masticatories and dyestuffs'. In SK. Jain (Ed). *Glimpses of Indian Ethnobotany,* 180–190.

Borthakur, SK,1997. 'Plants in the folklore and folk life of the Karbis (Mikirs) of Assam'. In SK. Jain (Ed): *Contribution to Indian ethnobotany* pp. 169-178, Scientific Publishers, Jodhpur.

Borthakur, SK and N. Goswami, 1995. 'Herbal remedies from Dimasa of Kamrup district of Assam in North-eastern India'. *Filoterabia* 66: 333-339.

Chauhan, AS. 1983. 'Dwindling taxa of Meghalaya', In SK. Jain and PR. Rao (Eds): *An Assessment of Threatened Plants of India*, pp. 142-145. Botanical Survey of India, Howrah, West Bengal.

Chowdhuri, SK.2000. 'Ethnobotany', In D. Mitra, J Guha; and SK. Chowdhuri (Eds): *Studies in Botany*, pp. 855–867, Vol. 2, 7th edn, Manai Press, Kolkata.

Das, S., PK. Dutta and BK Dutta. 2002. 'Ethnobotanical studies of Barak Valley, Assam. India'. In MK. Bhattacharjee, M. Dutta Choudhury and PB. Majumdar (Eds). *Bio Diversity of Assam and its Conservation.* Department of Botany, Karimganj College, Karimganj, Assam.

Dutta, BK. and PK. Dutta. 2005. 'Potential of ethnobotanical studies in N.E India. An overview', *Indian Journal of Traditional Knowledge.* 4,1: 7-14 .

Foster, GM, and BG Anderson, 1978. *Medical Anthropology.* New York Chichester Brisbane, Toronto: John Wiley and Sons.

Gogoi, P and CL Boissya, 1984. 'Information about a few herbal medicines used by the people of Assam (India) against Jaundice'. *Himalayan Research and Development* 2: 41–44.

Gunderson, L, and CS, Holling, 2002. 'Panarchy'. *Understanding Transformations in Human and Natural Systems*. Island Press, Washinton, D.C., USA.

Gupta, R. and KL. Chadha, 1995. 'Medicinal and aromatic plants in India'. In KL Chadha and R. Gupta (Eds): *Advances in Horticulture, Medicinal and Aromatic Plants*, pp.1-44, Malhotra Publishing House, New Delhi.

Hooker, JD. 1872-1897. 'The Flora of British India'. Volume I-VII. London: L. Reeve and Co.

Hughes, Charles C 1968. 'Ethnomedicine'. *International Encyclopedia of the Social Sciences*. Vol. 10. London: Crowell Collier and Macmillan Inc.

Jain, SK and RR. Rao.1977. *A Handbook of Field and Herbarium Methods*. New Delhi: Today and Tomorrow's Printers and Publishers.

Jain, SK. 1981. *Glimpses of Indian Ethnobotany*. pp. 365 Oxford and IBH.

Jain, SK. 1999. *Dictionary of Ethno Veterinary Plants in India*. Deep Publications, New Delhi.

Jain, SK. 1991. *Dictionary of Indian Folk Medicine and Ethnobotany*. Deep Publications, New Delhi.

Rout, Jayashree: L. Albert Sajem, and Minaram Nath. 2010. Traditional medicinal knowledge of the *Zeme (Naga)* tribe of North Cachar Hills District, Assam on the treatment of diarrhoea. *Assam University Journal of Science and Technology: Biological and Environmental Sciences* 5,1 : 63-69.

Kala, CP; PP Dhyani, and BS. Sajwan, 2006. 'Developing the medicinal plant's sector in Northern India: Challenge and opportunities'. *Journal of Ethnobiology and Ethnomedicine*, 2: 1-15.

Kanjilal, UN.; PC. Kanjilal, and A. Das, 1934-1940. *Flora of Assam*, Vol. I-IV. (Government of Assam, Shillong, India), Avon Book Company, Delhi.

Lalramnghinglova, H. 2000. 'Ethnobotany: A Review'. *Ethnobotany and Medicinal Plants of Indian Subcontinent*. Scientific Publishers, India.

Olsson, P, and C. Folke, 2001. 'Local ecological knowledge and institutional dynamics for ecosystem management: A case study of Lake Rachen watershed, Sweden', *Ecosystems* 4:85-104.

Pandi, KP., M. Ayyanar, and S. Ignacimuthu. 2007. 'Medicinal plants used by Malasar tribes of Coimbatore district, Tamil Nadu'. *Indian Journal of Traditional Knowledge*. 6, 4: 579.

Pareek, SK. 1996. 'Medicinal Plants in India: Present status and future prospects'. In *PL. Gautam et. al. (Eds): Prospects of Medicinal Plants*, pp. 5-14, Indian Society for Plant Genetic Resources, New Delhi.

Prakash, JW., RD. Anpin, AN. Asbin, C. Williams, GS. Regini, K. Bensar, R. Rajeev, S. Kiruba, S. Jeeva, and SSM. Das, 2008. 'Ethnomedicinal plants used by Kani tribes of Agasthiyarmalai Biosphere Reserve, Southern Western Ghats'. *Indian Journal of Traditional Knowledge*. 7, 3 : 410.

Pretty, JN. 2003a. *Agri-Culture: Reconnecting People, Land, and Nature*, pp. 8-16, Earthscan Publication Ltd, London, UK.

Pretty, JN. 2003b. 'Social capital and the collective management of resources'. *Science*, 302:1912-1914.

Sajem, AL and K. Gosai, 2006. 'Traditional use of medicinal plants by the Jaintia tribes in North Cachar Hills district of Assam, Northeast India. *Journal of Ethnobiology and Ethno Medicine* 2:33.

Sengupta, S. 2013. Anthropological studies on the people of North Eastern India. *The Indian Journal of Anthropology* 1, 1: 167-184.

Singh, AP., L. Gogoi, and J. Sebastian, 2015. 'The seasonality of butterflies in a semi-evergreen forest: Gibbon Wildlife Sanctuary, Assam, North-eastern India'. *Journal of Threatened Taxa,* 7,1: 6774-6787.

Singh, R.K., and AK. Sureja, 2006a. 'Community knowledge and sustainable natural resource management: Learning from *Monpa* tribe of Arunachal Pradesh', *TD: The Journal for Transdisciplinary Research in South Africa*, Northwest University, Norway, 2,1:73-102.

Singh, RK. and AK. Sureja, 2006b. 'Dynamics of traditional knowledge and prior informed consent of conservators of the indigenous biological diversity of Northeast India'. Paper presented in a *UGC sponsored National Seminar on Natural Resource and Tribal Community in North Eastern India on 7-8th February 2006* at Jawaharlal Nehru College, Pasighat, Arunachal Pradesh, India.

Syiem, D., B. Kharbuli B., DG. Das, I. Nongkhlaw D. Tharnar, G. Marngar, H. Synga, H. Kayang, B. Myrbon, YSH. Yobin, and DRM Buarn, 1999. 'Medicinal plants and herbal medicine : A case study in Meghalaya'. In B. Kharbuli, D. Syiem and Kayangh (Eds): *Biodiversity Northeast India Perspectives.* North Eastern Biodiversity Research Cell, NEHU, Shillong.

Takhtajan, AL. 1988. *Floristic Regions of the World.* Bishen Singh Mahendra Pal Singh, Dehradun (India), pp. 522.

Tamuli, P. and R. Saikia, 2004. 'Ethno-medico botany of the Zeme (Naga) tribe of North Cachar Hills District of Assam'. *Indian Journal of Traditional Knowledge.* 3, 4 : 430-436.

Tiwari, KC, R. Majumdar, and S. Bhattacharjee. 1979. 'Folklore medicine from Assam and Arunachal Pradesh (district Tirap)'. *International Journal of Crude Drug Research* 17: 61–67.

World Health Organisation Media Centre, 2008. *Traditional Medicine*, WHO, Geneva.

Yinegar, H. and D. Yewhalaw, 2007. 'Traditional medicinal plant knowledge and use by local healers in Sekoru District, Jimma Zone, Southwestern Ethiopia'. *Journal of Ethnobiology and Ethnomedicine.* 3: 24.

Chapter - 15

Ethnomedicinal Uses of *Ficus L.* in Assam

—*Priya Dhungana, Purnima Devi, and S.K. Borthakur*

Introduction

Knowledge of plants known by the tribals is important not just for themselves, but for the wider world. An example is Curare, from the Brazilian vine *Chondrodendron tomentosum* Ruiz and Pav., use as a hunting poison originally, but it contains tubocurarine which is now essential in surgery as a muscle relaxant. Another one is *Rauvolfia serpentina* (L.) Benth. ex Kurz, in India it was employed for centuries to treat mental disorders and insomnia, nowadays it provides the tranquiliser reserpine (Maheshwari, 1987). So, it is important to collect and document the information from tribal people before it is lost forever.

In India, research on ethnomedicine and other fields was initiated by Janaki Ammal (1956) while working in Botanical Survey of India. The study of ethnobotany was started during 1960 by Jain who is known as the "Father of Indian Ethnobotany" among different tribes of India including Northeastern Region of India (Jain and Borthakur, 1980; Jain and Dam, 1979).

Assam is one of the eight states of North-eastern India inhabited by many tribes using plants for different health problems. *Ficus* species are commonly known as "dimoru" in Assam is used by the local tribes for the treatment of various ailments. Therefore, the present study aims to document the ethnomedicinal uses of *Ficus* species by different tribes of Assam to know the potentiality of these species for further pharmacological works and utilisation to the benefit of mankind.

Methodology

A field survey was conducted during 2010-12 for the collection of widespread species of *Ficus* and data for enumeration. The information is based on the unstructured interview, discussion with local people and by personal observation of the authors. Voucher specimens were preserved in the form of herbarium as per standard field and herbarium technique (Jain and Rao, 1977) and submitted to Department of Botany, Gauhati University. The standard methods of ethnobotanical studies were followed which were undertaken by several researchers (Martin, 1995; Gupta, 1995; Jain, 1995; Mudgal, 1995; Rao and Hajra, 1995; Verma *et al.*, 2012).

Result

Table 15.1: Use of Ficus in Medicinal Preparations

Name of Plant	*Habitat*	*Local name*	*Part used*	*Type of Disease*	*Uses*
F. benga-lensis L.	Tree	*Bor*	Bark, Hanging aerial Root	Leucorrhoea, antiemetic, cuts and wounds, joint pains.	Bark powder use on vagina for curing leucorrhoea. The hanging roots are antiemetic. The paste prepared from the bark is applied to cuts and wounds and joint pains.
F. hispida L.	Shrub	*Khohota dimoru*	Root, Leaves, Latex	Diabetes, Liver ailments (jaundice), stomach diseases and inflammation.	Exudates from root taken in diabetes. Curry prepared from the leaf is taken in Liver ailments (jaundice). Leaves are also used for stomach problems. Latex is used for inflammation.
F. racemosa L.	Tree	*Jagya dimaru*	Fruits, Latex, Leaves, Roots	Diabetes, Mumps, liver and respiratory disorders. Carious tooth	Boiled fruits are given in diabetes. Applying of latex on the affected area while suffering from Mumps. Leaves used in the treatment of liver and respiratory disorders. Roots are used in carious tooth
F. religiosa L.	Tree	*Ahot*	Bark, Roots	Relieve pain during childbirth and wounds. Carious tooth, gonorrhea, liver disorders and boils	Bark decoction with a pinch of rock-salt is given to women after childbirth to relieve pain. Bark Ash with coconut oil on wounds. The bark is used in carious tooth, gonorrhea, liver disorders and boils. Roots are also used in carious tooth.

(Cont'd...)

F. rumphii Blume	Tree	*Jori*	Bark, Fruits	Eczema and ringworm. Asthma	Dried bark ash with coconut oil in eczema and ringworm. Fruits used in asthma.
F. hirta Vahl	Shrub	*Khongal dimoru*	Fruits	Cuts/Wounds	Fruits are used in cuts and wounds.
F. elastica Roxb.	Tree	*Rubber gach*	Bark, Root	Asthma and chest pain	Its bark and root powder is medicinal in a cough, asthma and chest pain.
F. benjamina L.	Shrub	*Sil bor*	Latex, Leaves	Eye diseases and wounds	Latex is used in eye diseases and leaves in wounds.
F. auriculata Lour.	Tree	*Athua dimaru*	Bark	Skin diseases and as a blood purifier.	Bark used in all types of skin diseases and its juice is used as a blood purifier.
F. virens Ait.	Tree	*Jori pakori*	Fruits	Anti-emetic	Fruits used in vomiting.

This study was carried out in districts of Upper Assam, India. This study had brought to light 10 common *Ficus* species which are used in medicinal preparations as claimed by the villagers/local healers to cure a number of ailments without any side effects (Table 15.1). During the survey, it was observed that for curing different ailments, the use of above ground plant parts was higher than the underground plant parts. Of the plant parts used, roots and barks (25 per cent each) are used in the majority of cases, followed by fruits (20 per cent) than by leaves and latex (15 per cent each) which contributed least in the medicinal usage. Most of the plant parts utilised were of trees (7) while only 3 plant species are of shrubs. The status of *Ficus* species according to percentage of treatment of diseases was also evaluated and it was found that *F. religious* contributed most in the medicinal formulations with the ability of curing six different types of diseases such as childbirth, wounds, carious tooth, gonorrhoea, liver ailments and boils followed by *F. racemosa,* used in the treatment of five diseases (diabetes, mumps, liver disorder, respiratory and carious tooth) and then by *F. bengalensis* and *F. hispida* with four diseases each reported to be cured such as leucorrhoea, cuts and wounds, joint pains, antiemetic and diabetes, liver ailments, stomach disease, inflammation respectively; *F. rumphii* reported to cure three different diseases such as skin disease, asthma, joint pains and; *F. auriculata* (skin disease and blood purifier), *F. benjamina* (eye disease and wounds) and least by *F. elastica* (respiratory disorder), *F. virens* (antiemetic) and *F. hirta* (cuts and wounds). Also, *Ficus* species was mostly reported for the treatment of cuts and wounds followed by liver ailments, joint pains, respiratory disorders and then by anti-emetic, diabetes, carious tooth, skin problems and least for the treatment of leucorrhoea, stomach disorders, mumps, childbirth, gonorrhoea, boils, ringworm, eye diseases, inflammation and blood purifier.

Discussion

In Assam, there are many widespread *Ficus* species locally known as "Dimoru" and used by the common people for various ailments. It is important to mention that, in the course of the survey, species of *Ficus* was found to be used for some gynae-related problems also. *F. bengalensis* is reported to be used for curing leucorrhea and *F. religiosa* for the relieve of pain during childbirth. *F. religiosa* is also found to be used for the treatment of gonorrhea, a sexually transmitted disease. The local people have a close relationship with the environment and have developed an indigenous knowledge of environmental protection as well as biodiversity conservation. It has been also reported by Buragohain (2011) that *F. racemosa* is used in the treatment of diabetes among the ethnic communities of Tinsukia district of upper Assam. During the study, it was observed that all the plant parts (leaves, fruits, latex, root, and barks) are used in various ailments and also, *F. racemosa* is reported to be the most useful plant according to the maximum number of plant parts used. Along with bark of *F. bengalensis*, fruits of *F. hispida* are also reported to be used by local communities around the Mayong region of Northeast India for curing leucorrhoea (Kalita *et al.*, 2011). Although species of *Ficus* are regarded as skin allergens, especially the latex is regarded as a serious eye irritant, but during the study, this belief is proven to be wrong as latex of *F. benjamina* found to use in treating eye diseases.

Conclusion

As the years are passing by, a gap is being built between the new generation and the age-old knowledge of ethnobotany. From the above study on the ethnomedicinal potentiality of *Ficus* species by the people of Assam, it can be concluded that the gathered information can be used for carrying out further pharmacological works especially that of the latex of the genus for the utilisation to the benefit of mankind.

References

Buragohain, J., 2011. 'Ethnomedicinal plants used by the ethnic communities of Tinsukia District of Assam, India'. *Recent Research in Science and Technology*. 3, 9: 31-42.

Gupta, SP., 1995. 'Study of plants during ethnological research among the tribals'. In SK. Jain (Ed): *A Manual of Ethnobotany*, pp. 9, Jodhpur; Scientific Publishers.

Jain, SK., 1995. 'Ethnobotany- Its scope and various sub-disciplines'. In SK. Jain (Ed.): *A Manual of Ethnobotany*, pp. 270. Jodhpur; Scientific Publishers.

Jain, SK and N. Dam, 1979. 'Some ethnobotanical notes from North Eastern India'. *Economic Botany*. 33, 1:52-56.

Jain, SK, and RR. Rao. 1977. *A Handbook of Field and Herbarium Methods*, New Delhi; Today and Tomorrow's Printers and Publishers.

Jain, SK, and SK. Borthakur, 1980. 'Ethnobotany of the Mikirs of India'. *Econ Bot*. 34, 3:264-272.

Janaki Ammal, EK., 1956. 'Introduction to the subsistence economy of India'. In LT. William Jr. (Ed.): *Man's Role in Changing Face of the Earth*. pp. 324-335. Chicago; University of Chicago Press.

Kalita, JC., B. Mahanta and A. Haque. 2011. 'An ethnomedicinal study on the medicinal plant of Mayong circle, Assam (India) used in leucorrhoea and assessment of the antifungal activity of *Solanum torvum* on *Candida albicans*'. *International Journal of Science and Advanced Technology*. 1, 5:177-184.

Maheshwari, JK., 1987. 'Interdisciplinary approaches in ethnobotany'. In SK. Jain (Ed.): *A Manual of Ethnobotany,* pp. 23-32, Jodhpur; Scientific Publisher.

Martin, G., 1995. *Ethnobotany: A 'People and Plants' Conservation Manual*, pp. 268, London; Chapman and Hall.

Mudgal, V., 1995. 'Recent ethnobotanical works on different states and tribes of India'. In SK. Jain (Ed.): *A Manual of Ethnobotany*, pp. 48, Jodhpur; Scientific Publishers.

Rao, RR, and PK. Hajra, 1995. 'Methods of research in ethnobotany'. In SK. Jain (Ed.): *A Manual of Ethnobotany,* pp. 28, Jodhpur; Scientific Publishers.

Verma, R., V. Parkash and D. Kumar, 2012. 'Ethnomedicinal uses of some plants of Kanag Hill in Shimla, Himachal Pradesh, India'. *International Journal of Research in Ayurveda and Pharmacy.* 3, 2: 319-323.

Chapter - 16

An Emic Perspective on Health and Sickness: The Minyongs

—*Maitreyee Sharma*

Introduction

Health and sickness are the social and biological concerns of human since its evolution. The concept of health is not merely biological, but to a significant extent socio-cultural, therefore, the concept varies from one cultural group to another. As a result, the Anthropological studies focus on local contexts where health and sickness are recognised and responded in their cultural representations. The definitions of 'health' seem evolved over time. The early definitions, however, focused on the theme of the body's ability to function; health was seen as a state of normal function that could be disrupted from time to time by disease. Then, in 1948, WHO proposed a definition that incorporating and linking health to well-being, in terms of "physical, mental, and social well-being, and not merely the absence of disease and infirmity". However, this definition was criticised as being very broad so in 1984 WHO revised this definition of health giving more importance to the dynamics of resiliency and defined it as "the extent to which an individual or group is able to realise aspirations and satisfy needs, and to change or cope with the environment. Health is a resource for everyday life, not the objective of living; it is a positive concept, emphasising social and personal resources, as well as physical capacities". According to Susser (1973), the term 'sickness' refers to socially and culturally held conceptions of health conditions and discomfort. It is the subjective experience of symptoms and suffering, which motivates changes in behaviour with a sociologically recognised meaning.

The tribes of North-East India need special attention in the domain of health and disease. This is because of two important reasons; firstly, most of the tribes live in isolated and remote areas where modern healthcare facilities are not easily accessible and secondly, the growth rate of the tribes show much variation among themselves. In addition to these major reasons, lack of personal hygiene and ignorance towards causative agents of sickness are factors that need immediate concern and research as well as dissemination of results to the concerned populations.

Materials and Methods

The Minyong is one of the tribes within the broader framework of the Adis of Arunachal Pradesh. They inhabit a large part of the Central, West, and South-Eastern Siang district of Arunachal Pradesh. They belong to the Mongoloid stock and their dialect belongs to the Tibeto-Burman family and very similar to the dialect of the Mishings of Assam (Taid, 2012). They are believed to be the descendants of the *Abo-Tani* (*Abo*-Father; *Tani*- Man) (Roy, 1960).The Minyongs believe that they have originated from *Pedong* (rain) *Ane* (mother); (Srivastava, 1990). Their oral narratives (*abang*) contain references to their southward migration from the Indo-Tibetan border.

The present chapter is based on the fieldwork conducted among the Minyongs of village Mori, West-Siang district of Arunachal Pradesh. Data are collected by interviewing several elder members of both the genders, individuals who have recently recovered from certain illness and one medicine-men (*Miri*), regarding their perception of health and sickness. The local informants neither practice nor prescribe the indigenous medicines and systems among the villagers, however, use this knowledge and information for their own requirement whenever necessary. To substantiate certain findings, a case-study method is applied. The researcher has used case study design for a number of reasons. The researcher chose this method particularly because the concepts of health and sickness are though biological but to a greater extent psycho-social. Thus, very much cultural as well as based on personal experiences. It is a study of the phenomenon, which focuses on specific instances that are cases and shades light of a phenomenon, which is a process, events, persons or things of interest to the researcher (Tuckman, 1994).

Result and Discussion

Concept of Health and Sickness among the Minyongs

Among the Minyongs, if an individual can perform its duties and day-to-day activities normally without any suffering are considered healthy. According to them, sickness (*kinam*) not merely refers to physical diseases but also mental illness and ailments. However, they relate health and sickness with the age of an individual. They believe that the youths possess warm blood with a lot of strength for which they are physically strong and do not fall sick easily. As one age, the warmth of the blood decreases due to which physical strength decreases and the risk of falling sick gradually increases. In the case of children, if the child is unable to walk or play properly from the second year (*ote-dugrik*) is taken seriously and considered physically weak. According to the villagers, the God, known as *Doini-Taleng*, is a powerful agency of causing sickness and ultimately death. It is he who decides at what time a man would die and which disease would be responsible for his death. He also assigns a particular spirit the responsibility of killing an individual with the such and such disease. When *Doini-Taleng* decides to do so, nothing can prevent the death of the intended person.

Causes of Illness

The Minyongs believe that they are surrounded by numerous spirits who play significant roles in the everyday affairs of their life. These spirits are both malevolent and benevolent. Some of them are considered very powerful and so people propitiate them so that their lives are free of troubles and sickness. The *urom* are considered as very influential spirits, which causes various diseases to the individuals possessed by them. The sacrifices after the consultation of the *Miri* may range from a single egg to a *Mithun* (esho). The anger of the spirits is considered the most important cause of death (*shinam*). Trespassing the territory of the spirits, accidental destroying of the spirits' abode in the jungles and in water are considered the prime causes of arousing the anger of the spirits and the spirits then take revenge of such destruction and interference by inflicting diseases and deformities to the convicted individuals. The individuals who had unnatural deaths like accident, suicide and women who died during childbirth become malevolent spirits and try to inflict various diseases to the living beings when angry or when need some kind of propitiation.

On asking why the spirits inflict human beings with diseases, one of the villagers narrated one of the folktales quite common among them, which answers my question. One of their folk tales states that- there were two very close friends-Tako and Tani. Tako was a spirit and Tani was a human being. Tako was benevolent as well as very innocent whereas Tani was very clever and he used to befool Tako whenever gets a chance. One day Tako approached Tani and said that his own fowls and pigs make irritable sounds due to which he could not sleep at night. On hearing this,

Tani immediately gave him a solution by stating that Tako should throw the animals down the hill. Next day Tako did accordingly but Tani was hiding behind the hill to collect the thrown animals. Next day Tani's son smeared the fat of the pigs thrown by the Tako and looked very fair and handsome. Tako on seeing such a sudden change asked Tani about the secret. Tani, as usual, to befool Tako said that he kept his son inside a basket for one night and covered with banana (*ekkam*) leaves. Then he poured boiling water over his face. Tako as usual believing Tani did the same with his son but next day he found his son dead inside the basket. Tako could not forget Tani's treachery and till today he takes revenge in various forms and happy to kill as many as Tani's children, i.e. the Minyongs.

The *epom* are another group of spirits who are always harmful to human beings. According to the Minyong legends, the *epom* were once very friendly to them but when the Minyongs became an expert in weaving various material culture and crafts, the *epom* became jealous and started making the trees their abode. These spirits, according to the Minyongs, are responsible for kidnapping individuals as well as responsible for inflicting night blindness and other eye infections. When someone is possessed by the *epom* spirits are tried to be propitiated with fowls (*perok*) and pigs (*ekk*) and by striking big trees. If the *epom* is pleased, the missing man returns to the family and if the man never returns then it is inferred that he has been eaten by the *epom*.

There are malevolent spirits that reside on the banks of the rivers and streams known as *asi among uyu*. They are thought to be responsible for causing paralysis. When someone is paralyzed, the spirit is offered with pigs rather than *Mithun* because the Minyongs believe that *asi among uyu* hate *Mithun*. After sacrificing and offering the pig to the spirit, the meat is offered to the paralyzed individual by the *Miri*. But this spirit according to the version of the *Miri* is very difficult to please and propitiate and very often kills the inflicted individual gradually.

In addition to these three kinds of spirits, there are also some other spirits which are responsible for causing common illness. A spirit known as *shikom tanom* is thought to cause swelling of the lower limbs. To prevent the occurrence of such edema, a fowl is killed and left somewhere on the way. It is the soul of the fowl that the spirit responsible is desirous of. If the *Miri* is not readily available; then any of the family members can offer the sacrifice to the spirit in the jungle.

Yet another spirit-*meju meya,* which live in small streams in the forest, inflict diarrhoea and body injuries. To propitiate them, a bamboo basket is filled with paddy husk and a bone of pig or *Mithun* and kept at the bank of the nearby stream. After that, it is assumed that the spirit eats the offered things and releases the ailing person.

Guming soying is another spirit causes swelling of the eye and ultimate blindness. To propitiate it, a fowl is killed, wrapped with boiled rice in a leaf, kept in a container and placed above the fireplace on the *perap* shelf. This spirit resides within the house and rarely invokes its anger and causes evil effects. The swelling and severe irritation of the eye may occur due to the continuous and long-term exposure to the soot and smoke coming out of the fireplace (*meram*) which keeps on emitting most of the time.

Another, prominent spirit-*nyine nyipak* is regarded to stay in the Granary (*kumsung*). This spirit is thought to cause stomach pain and vomiting immediately after meals. To relieve the pain, a fowl is killed and rice and *apong* are placed at the wheels fixed below the entrance of the granary. If still pain continues then the offerings are kept on the floor of the granary. However, if the *Miri* by trance comes to know that *nyine nyipak* is not responsible for the sickness then he instructs the family members to collect certain bamboo extracts and herbal parts and then he prescribes the required doses of the medicines to the sick.

Case 1: Mr Jerang Tatin, 34 years, Male, cultivator

> Mr Tatin suddenly felt sick after having his morning meal with severe stomach pain and vomiting. His wife immediately collected the tuber of *kekir* (*Zingiber zerambet* L. Smith) and fed a small crushed piece to Mr Tatin with warm water. *Kekir* is very commonly used to cure stomach ache and vomiting in the Minyong society. But his troubles remained the same and so his wife with utter fear called Mr Siyom Mije who is a *Miri* by profession. He while diagnosing the sick immediately came to know that it is the anger of the spirit- *nyine nyipak.* The *Miri* sacrificed a fowl (*perok*) while chanting in spirit dialect (*uyu-agam*) and offered boiled rice and *apong* and kept these over the entrance of the granary or *kumsung.* After about one hour, Mr Tatin gradually recovered from his stomach troubles and offered the *Miri* with a packet of rice and *apong.*

Health Specialist and Diagnosing System

When someone in the family falls sick, the other family members immediately communicate and consult a shaman or the *Miri*. The *Miri* is the religious head as well as the priest of the community. While diagnosing a disease, a *Miri* goes into trance and utters certain unintelligible words, which is regarded as *uyu-agam* or spirit language. This is regarded as the conversation of the *Miri* with the spirit in their land (*tako merik*). If the concerned Spirit is pleased with him, it helps him in diagnosing the cause of the disease and prescribes a suitable sacrifice for its cure. If the spirit agrees to release the soul of the patient, he gets well, but if they do not, death is certain.

The main method of diagnosing diseases by *Miri* is divination. The most common method of divination is by the observation of the liver of a fowl. The *Miri* splits the stomach of the fowl as offered by the family members of the sick and takes out the liver delicately. He then divides it into two parts- one for divination of causes inside the village of the sick and another for divination outside the village. Various spots with various colours and magnitude denote different diseases and different spirits responsible for causing the disease. Accordingly, sacrifices should be offered for their cure.

Sometimes, but very rarely, when the disease shows fluctuating symptoms, a pig is killed for the purpose of divination. The liver of the pig is taken out and examined very carefully by the *Miri* and prescription depends on the condition of the liver and the inner skin of the patella of the pig. If the liver shows yellowish spots then the sick is suffering from jaundice. The condition of the patella skin refers to the spirit directly responsible for the sickness.

There is yet another simple and interesting method of divination practiced by the *Miri*. The *Miri* rubs dirt mixed with water on the body of the patient with the help of bamboo slice collects this dirt on a leaf and drinks it. The *Miri* then waits for some time to see the reaction of the dirt of the patient with his own body inside. If he vomits after sometimes, the patient may not survive for long but if the *Miri* remains normal without vomiting, the result is expected positive and the patient may get healed soon.

It is interesting that the *urom* is considered to cause barrenness and consecutive miscarriages in a woman in order to extract some sacrifice from the family concerned. *Oma tornam* sacrifice is performed to remove barrenness in a woman.

Case 2. Mrs Yamir Mije, female, 41 years, cultivator

Mrs Yamir Mije is a mother of one child. She conceived the child after 11 years of marriage and after her first child, she is unable to conceive further. It was her husband who for the first time thought of consulting a *Miri* to solve their problem of childlessness. On their consultation, the *Miri* advised them to organise a sacrifice typically meant for curing barrenness of women-*oma tornam*. In this sacrifice, the *Miri* divined with the help of pebbles to identify the spirit responsible. He took nine pebbles in the hollow of the two hands and chanted over them certain unintelligible words. After that, he thrown the pebbles on the ground and halved the pebbles and removed the odd and even pebbles from each group. The remainder of the pebbles of the two halves showed the cause of her barrenness. In their case, *urom* was said to be appeased with the sacrifice of a fowl. After sacrificing the fowl, the *Miri* chopped off the legs of the fowl and waved them over the abdomen and reproductive parts of the woman concerned. The *Miri* was then remunerated with the flesh of the sacrificed fowl, a packet of rice and *apong*. The result is expected to follow immediately. However, in their case, she conceived after 8 months of this sacrificial ritual.

Spontaneous abortion or *ori* is also considered an act of *urom*. During painful parturition or when childbirth does not take place easily, the family members sacrifice a dog or a fowl to appease the *urom* responsible-*nippong*. Sometimes a *Miri*, if on hand, is called upon to do the ritualistic sacrifice. The Minyongs believe that the spirits of women who die during childbirth become *nippong uyu* and when needs propitiation induces troubles during the childbirth.

Case 3. Mr Tayo Tatin, male, 24 years, cultivator

> Mr Tayo Tatin is a father of two children. When his wife suffered from terrible complications during her third childbirth, he along with the family members consulted a *Miri* during her delivery. The *Miri* entered into a trance and advised him to sacrifice a fowl immediately to appease the *nippong uyu* responsible for obstruction of the delivery passage. However, unfortunately, according to Mr Tatin, the anger of the *uyu* could not be reduced and appeased and the baby was born dead. Had the *urom* appeased, the baby would have survived. The stillborn baby (*oripe*) was then entered into a scooped out pumpkin by him and hang on a tree branch of an unfrequented jungle in the belief that the *nippong uyu* would see the result and would not do this again in their life.

There are certain herbal medicines known by almost every Minyong of the village which is used to cure certain commonly occurring health problems like a snake bite, stomach ache, vomiting, diarrhoea, jaundice, fever, cold, nose-bleeding, toothache and bone fractures.

- *Solanum nigrum* L (Solanaceae)-*Bangko*-Leaves, roots, and stem- Leaves are boiled in water and the extract is given to diarrhea and malaria patients for four to five days. The juice of the crushed roots of *Bangko* is given to the malaria patient. Warm leaves are put over the eye to cure eye infections.
- *Zanthoxylum rhetsa* DC- *Onger*- Leaves and fruits- Leaves are dried and crushed and then applied on the tooth to get relief from a toothache. The fruit is eaten raw in large quantity for inducing abortion. The juice is also given to the jaundice patients.
- *Zingiber cassumunar* (Zingiberaceae)-*Kekir*- Tuber- the extract of the tuber is given to get relief from stomach ache, vomiting as well as from a cough. Moreover, the tuber is cooked along with other vegetables and given to the mother for the reduction of post-delivery pain.
- *Annanus comosus* (Bromeliaceae) - *Anaros/Tako*- Fruit- Women use the fruit as abortifacient, as natural fertility controlling agent.
- *Coptis teeta* (Ranunculaceae)- *Ringko/Mishimi teeta*- Roots and leaves- The roots are crushed and powdered after drying. Then the powder is boiled with water and administered to the malaria patient. The extract of the leaves along with raw papaya is used by women as abortifacient.
- *Aristolochia indica* L.-*Hinger*-Whole plant- The whole plant parts are grinded and consumed immediately after snake bite for three to five days twice daily.

Conclusion

Thus, like every other society, the Minyongs of Arunachal Pradesh also have its own perspective on health and sickness and the traditional knowledge to struggle sickness and to remain healthy. They try to challenge sickness and disease in their own ways by consulting a *Miri* or sometimes by ingesting herbal plants found locally by them. Different parts of plants are used to cure various commonly occurring ailments like stomachache, toothache, bone fractures, cough and cold, jaundice, diarrhoea, eye infections and also snake bite. They attribute sickness solely to the anger of spirits. However, any normal individual cannot achieve the status of a *Miri*. A *Miri* generally shows the signs of going into trance and utters spirit language/ *uyu-abang* during the period of trance from his early childhood and goes about chanting these in the village. He is believed to be spirit-possessed and can generate secret relationships with the *uyus* responsible for diseases. The *uyus* then tell him to appease with appropriate offerings and sacrifice in order to release the individual. However, not all the diseases can be cured by such offerings and sacrifices. Perhaps, their immense faith on the *Miri* i.e. psychological satisfaction after performing offerings and sacrifice is the main power that heals their sickness to a larger extent and most often.

References

Roy, S., 1960. *Aspects of Padam Minyong Culture*, Directorate of Research; Government of Arunachal Pradesh.

Srivastava, LR., 1990. *Social Organisation of the Minyongs*. Directorate of Research; Government of Arunachal Pradesh.

Susser, M., 1973. *Causal Thinking in the Health Sciences*. New York; Oxford University Press.

Taid, TR., 2012. 'The Mising and their speech', In JJ. Kuli (Ed): *The Misings: Their History and Culture*, Dibrugarh; Kaustubh Prakashan.

Tuckman, PH.,1994. *Conducting Educational Research*. 4th Edition. Philadelphia; Harcourt Brace College Publishers.

World Health Organisation. 1948. 'Constitution of the World Health Organisation'. In *World Health Organisation: Basic Documents*. 45th Edition. Geneva; World Health Organisation.

World Health Organisation. 1984. *Health Promotion: A Discussion Document*. 1984. New York.

Chapter - 17

Knowledge and Use of Medicinal Plants by Khasi, Garo, and Karbis of North East India

—H.N. Dhungana, K.N. Barua and P.K. Hazarika

Introduction

From the time immemorial human beings have used the plant species for the treatment of different types of diseases. Knowledge of Indian medicinal plants can be traced back from the Vedic period. North Eastern Region of India is endowed with a rich wealth of medicinal plants, a remarkable bio-cultural diversity and an enormous wealth of indigenous knowledge accumulated over long past and passed down from generation to generation with oral tradition. Due to lack of documentation and introduction of modern technologies the preservation of indigenous knowledge is at risk. It is also rapidly being lost, as the ecosystem is degraded, traditional cultures and communities disintegrated or they are moving towards modern culture. However, the traditional system of medicine plays a very prominent role in healthcare system of the rural people. Like all other indigenous tribal communities of North Eastern region, Khasi, Garo and Karbi tribes also are closely associated with nature. Due to this association, they were able to develop their own traditional knowledge on the use of plants for various ailments.

Study of plants used by various tribes of North East India have been carried out from time to time by several workers such as Borthakur (1976), Jain and Borthakur (1980), Rao and Neogi (1980), Rao (1981), Tiwari *et al.* (1992,1993), Pandey *et al.* (1996), Lalramnghinglova (1996), Singh *et al.* (1996), Choudhury and Neogi (1999), Barua *et al.* (2003), Nath and Maiti (2003), Baruah *et al* (2006), Das *et al.* (2006), Hynniewta and Kumar (2008) and others.

Previous ethnobotanical study in this area

Biswas and Ahmed (1987) carried out sporadic ethnobotanical studies on medicinal and vegetable wealth in some plants available in the area. Sharma and Sharma (2010) also documented ethnomedicines of Sonapur, Kamrup District, Assam which is very near to the present study site.

Study Site

The present study was conducted during 2010-12, in Ri-Bhoi district of Meghalaya and Kamrup district of Assam bordering bordering Ri-Bhoi district, which extends from 91° 49' 53.1" E to 91° 55' 51.9" E and 25° 52' 58.5" N to 26° 06' 50.4" N. The area was preferred where three targeted tribes (Khasi, Garo, and Karbi) are inhabited nearby and the location is near the city or town. Fourteen villages namely Umlangpur, Nongthymmai, Umdow, Nongkhrah and Marngar (Khasi villages), Jorbil, Umpher, Rangsakuna, Maikhuli and Pillangkata (Garo villages), Ronghona, Sonaigaon, Aparikola and Morokdola (Karbi villages) were selected for the study.

Study Method

Periodical interview/discussion/meeting was organised with a key informant, elderly persons, women, and patient for collection of information on indigenous knowledge on plants found useful in herbal medicine, a way of drug preparation, doses, a method of administration and various medicinal recipes. Questionnaires were used for collecting the information. The assessment was made for attitudinal change among the target tribal groups towards traditional medical practices in the changing socio-economic situation due to the establishment of the primary health centre, construction of road and other developmental activities. Samples of unidentified plants were collected with their local name and subsequently identified properly with the help of available literature and ASSAM Herbarium, BSI, Shillong. Methods of botanical collection and herbarium techniques were followed as suggested by Jain and Rao (1977).

Results and Discussion

A total of 70 numbers of medicinal plants were documented and out of which 12 plant species were very commonly available on the road side or nearby houses in the study area (Table 17.1). These herbal medicines were used by the villagers for day-to-day therapeutically remedies and it has been observed that villagers of almost all groups were aware of the uses of these plants. Some plants were preserved by the local inhabitants for their healthcare (Table 17.2). Among the listed plant species *Phlogacanthus thyrsi floras, Bacopa monnieri, Clerodendrum colebrookianum, Houttuynia cordata, Paederia foetida, Aloe vera and Bryophyllum pinnatum* were planted in maximum households. Some traditional medicine men collect the medicinal plants from the field and prepare medicines for various ailments. Some plant extract and dried stem powder are prescribed for curing different diseases. However, their recipes are generally kept secret and proper identification of the used plant species is not easy from the dried materials. The younger generations are reluctant to learn the uses of traditional medicinal system from the elders, so information is not totally passed on to the successor. For better utilisation of the herbal drugs and save rich traditional sources of knowledge for the future generation, some conservational strategies are most essential. Possibilities of medicinal plants for livelihood opportunities need to be explored.

Table 17.1: Medicinal plants commonly available in the site

Botanical name	***Family***	***Local name***	***Uses***
Ageratum conyzoides L.	Asteraceae	*Myngai (Kh), Gondhua Bon (Ass)*	Leaf juice is used in cuts and wounds and also for removing hair lice.
Alternanthera sessilis(L.) R. Br. ex DC.	Amaranthaceae	*Raeaba (Kr), Matikanduri (Ass)*	Stem and leaf paste applied locally against snake bite.
Centella asiatica (L.) Urban	Apiaceae	*Kynbatmaina(Kh), Bormanimuni (Ass)*	Juice of the whole plant is used in dysentery, stomachache and eye infection.
Clerodendrum viscosum Vent.	Verbenaceae	*Loholaw (Kh), Samati (G) Dhopat tita (Ass)*	Juice of young leaves is used in dysentery. Leaf is also used in acidity and sprain.
Cuscuta reflexa Roxb.	Convolvulaceae	*Durimmel (G) Akashi lota (Ass)*	Plant juice is used in jaundice.
Lantana camara L.	Verbenaceae	*Dieng shopang khlien (Kh), Guphul (Ass)*	Leaf paste is used in skin diseases and also stops bleeding.
Leucas aspera Spreng.	Lamiaceae	*Chanrong aan (Kr), Thungkut (G)Doron (Ass)*	One drop of leaf juice is used as a drop, once daily for six days in sinusitis. Leaf juice is also given in skin eruptions and swelling.
Melastoma malabathricum L.	Melastomaceae	*Khakhuchi (Gr), Soh-khing (Kh), Phutkola (As)*	The leaf juice is mixed with rice water and taken for gastric pain. Leaf extract is also applied in dysentery and worm infestation in children.

(Cont'd...)

Mimosa pudica L.	Mimosaceae	*Smit-ship (Gr), Lajuki lota (As)*	Leaf juice with milk is taken for piles and boils.
Mikania micrantha kunth.	Asteraceae	*Jermapakistan (K)*	Leaf juice is used on cuts to stop bleeding.
Scoparia dulcis L.	Scoraphula-riaceae		Whole plant paste is applied to reduce a headache and giddiness.
Solanum nigram L.	Solanaceae	*Soh-ngang (Kh), Pharchingki (Kr) Lach kachi (Ass)*	Fruits are used in the intestinal worm.

Table 17.2: Plant preserved in Homestead garden for therapeutic uses

Botanical name	***Family***	***Local name***	***Uses***
Abroma augusta L.f.	Sterculiaceae		Leaf juice is applied for ringworm.
Aloe vera (L.) Burm. f.	Liliaceae	*Chalkuwari (Ass)*	Very good medicine for the burn. It is also good for skin.
Averrhoa carambola L.	Oxalidaceae	*Kordoi (Ass)*	Fruits are used for Jaundice.
Andrographis paniculata (Burm. f.) Wall. ex Nees	Acanthaceae	*Chirata*	The whole plant is used in a stomachache.
Azadirachta indica A. Juss.	Meliaceae	*Maha Neem*	Leaf is used against skin diseases and diabetes.
Bryophyllum pinnatum (Lam.) Oken	Crassulaceae	*Samjangi(G)*	Leaf paste is used for blister, cuts, and wound.
Clerodendrum colebrookianum Walp.	Verbenaceae	*Tongama (G) Nephaphu (Ass)*	Boiled leaves are used to control high blood pressure.
Hibiscus rosa-sinensis L.	Malvaceae	*Joba (Ass)*	Flowers are used in menstruation and urinary complications.
Murraya koenigii (L) Spreng.	Rutaceae	*Thengsakso (Kr), Narashingha (As)*	Leaves used in abdominal gripe, intestinal colic, and dysentery.
Nyctanthus bor tristis L.	Oleaceae	*Hewali (Kr), Sewali phul (As)*	Leaf juice is used in malaria. *a r -*
Ocimum sanctum L.	Lamiaceae	*Tiew lapongnai (Khasi)*	Leaf juice with honey is used for a cough.
Paederia foetida L.	Rubiaceae	*Rekang nemthu (Kr), Bhedailota (Ass)*	Leaf juice once daily after meal for a week is used in gastric problem.
Phlogocanthus thrysiflorus Nees.	Acanthaceae	*Ram bahak (Ass), Dieng-soh-kajut (Kh)*	Leaves are used as an expectorant in a cough, bronchitis, and asthma.

(Cont'd...)

Phyllanthus emblica L.	Euphorbia-ceae	*Bon bakeri (Gr), Amlokhi (Ass)*	Fruits are used in constipation and diabetes.
Pogostemon benghalensis (Burm.f.) Kuntze	Lamiaceae	*Suklati (Ass)*	Applied to stop bleeding.
Psidium guajava L.	Myrtaceae	*Madhuri aam (Ass)*	A bark decoction is taken for stomachache. Tender leaves used for a toothache.
Spondius pinnata (L.f.) Kurz	Anacardia-ceae	*Siming (Kr) Amora (Ass)*	Bark used in dysentery, urticaria, melaena and blood dysentery. Fruit used in diarrhea and cough.
Terminalia chebula Retz.	Combreta-ceae	*Marsang (Kh), Silikha (Ass)*	Root used in jaundice, fruit used in vomiting, constipation and fruit juice in a stomachache.
Houttuynia cordata Thunb.	Saururaceae	Ja-myrdoh (Kh) Machudori (G) Masundori (Ass)	A paste of leaves and roots took to cure dysentery. It also enhances appetite.
Bacopa monnieri (L.) Wettst.	Plantagina-ceae	Brahmi (Ass)	Used as brain tonic.

(Kh = Khasi, Kr = Karbi, G = Garo, Ass= Assamese).

Acknowledgment: The authors are thankful to the Director, Rain Forest Research Institute, Jorhat for providing facilities to carry out the present work. The authors are also thankful to village Headmen and informants for their assistance during the field work.

References

Barua, KN., IC. Barua and M. Das, 2003. 'Ethno botany of Rajbanshis of Assam', In JK. Maheshwari (Ed): *Ethno Botany and Medicinal Plants of Indian Sub-continent,* pp. 609-614, Jodhpur; Scientific Publisher.

Biswas, S and A. Ahmed, 1987. 'Ethnobotanical studies on some parts of Burnihat Valley, Assam and Meghalaya', *Indian Forester* 113, 9:634-639.

Borthakur, SK., 1976. 'Less known medicinal uses among the tribes of Karbi-Anglong (Mikir Hills), Assam', *Bulletin of the Botanical Survey of India,* 18, 1-4:166-171.

Chaudhury, D and B. Neogi, 1999. 'Ethnobotanical of Khasi and Chakma tribes of North East India'. *J. Econ. Tax. Bot.* 23, 2: 583-589.

Das, AK., BK. Dutta and GD. Sharma, 2006. 'Study of medicinal plants used by the different tribes and communities of Cachar District, Assam – 1'. *J. Econ. Tax. Bot.* 30 (Suppl.): 294-309.

Hynniewta, SR and Yogendra Kumar. 2008. 'Herbal remedies among the Khasi traditional healers and village folks in Meghalaya'. *Indian Journal of Traditional Knowledge* 7, 4: 581-586.

Jain, SK, and RR. Rao, 1977. *A Handbook of Field and Herbarium Methods*, New Delhi; Today and Tomorrow's Printers and Publishers.

Jain, SK, and SK. Borthakur, 1980. 'Ethnobotany of Mikirs of India'. *Econ. Bot.* 34, 3:264-272.

Lalramnghinglova, JH., 1996. 'Ethnobotany of Mizoram: A preliminary survey', *Journal. Econ. Taxon. Bot.* Additional Series 12: 439-459.

Nath, Ashish, and GG. Maiti. 2003. 'Ethnobotany of Barak Valley (Southern Assam) with special reference to folk medicine'. *J. Econ. Taxon. Bot.* 27, 4: 964-971.

Pandey, AK., HR. Bora and SC. Deka, 1996. 'An ethno-medico-botanical study of Golaghat district, Assam: Native plant remedies for Jaundice', *Journal. Econ. Taxon. Bot.* Additional Series 12: 344-349.

Rao, RR and B. Neogi, 1980. 'Observation of the ethnobotany of the Khasi and Garo tribes in Meghalaya (India)'. *J. Econ. Tax. Bot.* 1, 1-2: 157-162.

Rao, RR., 1981 'Ethno botany of Meghalaya: Medicinal plants used by Khasi and Garo tribes'. *Econ. Bot.* 35, 1: 4-9.

Sharma, R, and HK. Sharma, 2010. 'Ethno medicines of Sonapur, Kamrup District, Assam'. *Indian Journal of Traditional Knowledge,* 9, 1: 163-165.

Singh, J., TC. Bhuyan and A. Ahmed, 1996. 'Ethno botanical studies on the Mishing tribes of Assam with special reference to food and medicinal plants - I', *Journal. Econ. Taxon. Bot.* Additional Series 12: 350-356.

Tiwari, KC., BN. Sharma, RN. Majumder and G. Pandey, 1993. 'Studies on medicinal plants of Khasi and Jaintia Hills in North Eastern region of India'. *J. Econ. Tax. Bot.* 17, 2: 275-281.

Tiwari, KC., GC. Joshi, NK. Pandey and G. Pandey, 1992. 'Some rare folk tribal medicines from Garo Hills in North Eastern India'. *J. Econ. Tax. Bot. Addl. Ser.* 10: 319-322.

Chapter - 18

Traditional Pregnancy Care among the Thadou of Manipur

—Tonjam Joshila Chanu and M.C. Arunkumar

Introduction

Despite the amazing advancement in modern allopathic treatment in pregnancy, traditional healthcare practices have always been used by indigenous ethnics of the World, including the tribal people of India. Their knowledge for the traditional treatment of reproductive health especially pregnancy can be attributed to the abundance and rich diversity of medicinal plants in their habitat. Their wide knowledge of surrounding diverse ecology brings to work for their benefit in a very best way, among which ethnomedicine is one noticeable and valuable knowledge which need special attention. Generally, it is believed that childbirth is a normal component of life such as sexual maturation and pregnancy surrounded by cultural, social, ethical and religious considerations. The status of reproductive health is widely varied depending on the prevailing practices of the individual and community at large. The environmental factors and usage of traditional knowledge, beliefs and taboos are also responsible for determining the reproductive health status of any society. The knowledge of the intimate relationship between man and plants in his immediate surrounding has been passed mainly through tradition (Jain, 2004). This traditional knowledge about the use of naturally available herbs and their products has been transmitted through oral communication within the society and has been passed from generation to generation.

Tribes have their own culture and social practices to treat various illnesses. They have considered that the cause of illness or disease is related to his or her activities in society and to the environment where he or she is located. The disease cannot be seen as separate from is social-cultural-environmental context. It has been pointing out that in Rio Negro tribal society every event which occurs during the women's reproductive age is immediately inscribed in the totality of the socio-cultural environmental context.

Tribal communities possess a unique healthcare approach concerning the acceptance and rejection of modern medicine. They have retained much of their traditional healthcare during pregnancy and post-delivery period. The relationship between a tribal woman and traditional healthcare is based on trust, responsibility, charity, power, and respect from which she expects more than skill-based interventions as treatment (Ali, 1994). It is also observed that reproductive health of the tribal population is comprised of supernatural beliefs related to illness and treatment, the strong role of traditional medicine men or shamans, community involvement in disease control and treatment, mixed interventions of traditional and modern healthcare (Chaudhuri, 1994).

It has been observed from a recent study that there is a keen inclination among the tribal women towards modern medical facilities if accessible (Kumar, 2007; Chanu, 2010). WHO also recommends that some traditional medical resources, such as some medicinal plants could be used after an evaluation where the beneficial resources should be selected and those considered harmful to health should be discarded. Traditional tribal socio-religious practices also can be adversely affected their women's reproductive health as well as tribal's general health, such as alcohol consumption during pregnancy (Salehin, 2012).

In recent times with the increasing knowledge of life and culture of tribal communities, the social scientists are taking interest in ethnomedicinal studies. Many works have been reported, especially from among the rural and tribal communities of India. Dash and Dash (2003) have observed that although a large number of plant species as traditional medicines are dominant in the entire tribal society. Ray and Sharma (2005) have given a description of ethnomedicinal beliefs and practices prevalent among the Savaras, a Tribal community of Andhra Pradesh. Kumari (2006), gave an account on the concept of illness and disease and the application of folk medicine among the Sauras of Jharkhand.

India has the largest concentration of tribal in the world perhaps in Africa. According to the census 2001, as many as 84.33 million are classified as scheduled tribes (STs). North-East India is a land inhabited by more than 200 fascinating tribes. Different ethnic groups and tribal groups inhabit the region of northeast India. They all have their own culture and tribal tradition and all speak their own tribal languages. Tribes of Manipur which represent a unique feature of the land include at least 33 communities that originated from Tibetan-Burman tribal group Mongoloids. The present study was carried among the Thadou tribes of Saikul of Manipur and it is one of the recognised tribes of India in Manipur. They have been classified as New Kuki tribes and falls under the broad Tibeto-Burman linguistic stock spread over India's Northeastern region (Grierson, 1904). The Thadou tribe has enriched their culture and tradition with its plethora of folktales, songs, dance, and verses. Only a few studies (Sanglakpam *et.al.,* 2012; Devi, 2012) have carried out on the tribal of the state who utilises a number of medicinal plants available in surrounding area as treatment of various diseases. But the information on traditional knowledge on herbs used for reproductive health is meager in these populations.

About the Field Site

The present study broadly deals with the traditional knowledge regarding reproductive health among the Thadous, of Saikul town of Manipur. The study covered Thadou villages of Saikul town. The Thadous is an agrarian community; agriculture and farming are their most common form of socioeconomic organisation. They also practice other means of livelihood and work habitats such as hunting, gathering, weaving, etc. They are mostly Baptism in Christian religion and literacy rate is comparatively high among them. Looking at the ratio of literacy, female literacy rate is lesser than that of the male. There are four private high schools and one secondary school in this small town. Communication and transportation system with other places and Capital of State is easily available. There is one Primary Health Centre at the heart of the town. People have well acquaintance with the services of Health Centre. A recent study done by the author has found that 100 per cent of the pregnant women visited for antenatal care in Health Centre. Rapport was established before data collection. The data was collected from the local knowledgeable elderly persons mostly old women, who conduct delivery. They do not undertake their medical service as a vocation; they are mostly farmers and housewives. The medical service they have undertaken, though not free of charge but they performed on ethical grounds and noncommercial nature. The old woman was interviewed for recording the local names of plants parts used, the purpose of usage and the method of administration.

Traditional Knowledge in Thadou Community

Earlier, the Thadou society, the use of traditional medicines was predominant. But with time advent of modern medical facilities, the traditional medicine is losing its efficacy. Available evidence (Table 18.1) and (Table 18.2) indicates that traditional medicines are involved in providing reproductive healthcare. The use of traditional medicines for reproductive healthcare is due to subsisting mutual beliefs; they considered pregnancy and pregnancy-related problems as a natural occurrence. In the present study, some plants species, fouls and animal meats are being used for different reproductive health problems, especially during the pregnancy periods. The version of the villagers revealed that people have been shifting from traditional medicine from modern medicine system. This is due to the effectiveness or quick action and easy availability of modern medicines. Restriction and uses of certain plants and plants products for reproductive health have been highlighted in this chapter.

Table 18.1: Accepted items used by Thadou for Reproductive Health

English Name	*Local name/ locality*	*Purpose of use*	*Mode of use*
Ash guard	*Torbot/ Maipung*	To reduce white discharge	Soaked with cow milk and drink daily
Amla	*Heikru*	To reduce vaginal discharge	Mix with red sugar and drink it before food
	Shundari mana	To reduce vaginal itching	Boil with water and frequently
Banana plant	*Laphu*	To initiate lactation	Banana stem boil with water and make it as side dish food
Edible taro	*Yendem*	To initiate lactation and blood increase	Cook it as food curry
	Pan	For easy delivery	Cook it as food curry
Ginger	*Shing*	To regulate menstrual disorder	Boil with water or cooked with other vegetables
	Yembum mana	To initiate lactation	Cook it as food curry without oil
Pig/Cow tail	*Oak/Shan mamei*	Good for womb and increase blood after delivery	Cook it as food curry without oil
Honey	*Khoihee*	Good for initiate lactation	Applying it to nipples just after delivery
Water rice	*Chenghee/ Chabon*	Good for womb	Drink it before food

Table 18.2: Restricted items by the Thadou for reproductive health

English name	*Local name/ locality*	*Restricted period*	*Purpose for restriction*
Black rice	*Chakhou*	During Menstruation	Helps in skin darkening
Fruits	*Hei*	During Menstruation	Causes abdomen pain and disorder
Banana flower	*Laphou tharou/Naga*	During Menstruation	Causes less blood
Red meat	*Sha*	During Menstruation	Causes body pain and itching vaginal
Crab	*Waikhu*	During pregnancy	Causes Miscarriage
	Vailu	During early stage of pregnancy	Causes miscarriage and vaginal discharge
Beehives	*Khoira*	During pregnancy	Causes fever during delivery time
Pumpkin	*Mairen*	During breastfeeding	Causes less lactation

In spite of easily accessible of a modern facility, Thadou is still practicing some indigenous knowledge during menstruation and pregnancy period. They are keeping restriction of sex for three months after delivery. They kept straight legs while sitting during the delivery time so that it will heal the wounded portion very fast and keep the body in bright future in the later stage. Heavy things are not carried in the early stage of pregnancy but they are doing floor moping in a later stage as it will help in easy delivery. A pregnant woman is not allowed to attain a funeral because it causes the miscarriage. It is also a belief that during menstruation girls should not mingle with boys or men because it will cause illness in the womb. At the time of delivery, the woman takes bath with very hot water. This is continuing for about a week. After taking bath, hot boiled chicken soup is given to the woman. So that it will help the body for quick recovery. In olden days women were serving with black hen but now-a-days hen or cock is given. During the delivery time, women are given only the boil food without any chilies.

The present study is based on the data collected from the different villages around the Saikul Town. The local uses of plants/herbs, plant production, fouls and animal meats or parts are used in the family were elder women or experienced women stayed. But these people are easily availing the modern medicines nearby town or from the capital town of the State and it is also observed that new generations or young people are not interested this kind of treatment of traditional methods or indigenous practices. They did not know the social classes including the poor are giving up traditional health practices and turning to western bio-medicine (Shanker, 2009). However, restriction of certain indigenous practices is still guarded among the Thadou society irrespective of family income or status. Unfortunately, they do not keep any written records or books for this indigenous knowledge but transmitted orally down through the ages.

The observation reveals that the Thadou use leaves, roots, stem, and seed as medicinal preparation to use different reproductive health problems. On another hand, they are also restricted to use some of the plants and plants products and animal meats in order to prevent from the causes of reproductive health problems. Although the information collected from the elders and experienced women is not comparable with the modern medicines their efficacy is claimed to be high among the Thadous. Despite all factors, the Thadou are still using traditional medicines and indigenous practices, though the prevalence of this knowledge is waning.

Conclusion

The study reveals that the Thadou has vast knowledge about the ethnomedicinal uses of plants growing in their vicinity. The traditional healing system is based on the indigenous knowledge of local elders which has practiced on beliefs and customs related to health, specific to each locality and passed on from generation to generation by word of mouth. It is also confirmed that they make use of a surprisingly wide array of locally available flora and fauna. It has been well revealing in this study that the Thadou community has been changing at a certain pace along with their health seeking behaviour. The growing disinterest in the use of traditional medicines or indigenous knowledge among the younger generation will lead to the disappearance of this practice. Due to the process of urbanisation and cultural contact, wide spread of western medicines available in the State, there is a threat to the indigenous knowledge emerges gradually giving rise to a situation of medicinal pluralism. However, the study certainly points out that the traditional reproductive healthcare system still finds its meaning of survival in Thadou community. Therefore, there is urgent need to implement a revitalisation strategy for protecting the indigcnous from complete desertion.

References

Ali, A., 1994. 'Indigenous health practices among tribals. Relationship with prevalent disease'. In S. Basu (Ed): *Tribal Health in India*; pp. 130-150. New Delhi; Manak Publications Pvt. Ltd.

Chanu, Joshila., 2010. *A Study of Reproductive Health among the Meiteis, Muslims, and Tribal Population of Imphal East*. Unpublished ICSSR, New Delhi Sponsored Project Report. Anthropology Department; Manipur University.

Chaudhuri, B., 1994. 'Social and environmental dimensions of tribal health'. In S. Basu (Ed): *Tribal Health in India*; pp. 70-83. New Delhi; Manak Publications Pvt. Ltd.

Dash, B, and NC. Dash., 2003. 'Ethnobotany of Khonds of Ganjam'. In PK. Chand and SN. Patro (Ed): *Science for Society*. pp. 132-135, Bhubaneswar; ISCA Publication.

Devi, P and P. Suresh Kumar., 2012. 'Traditional, ethnic and fermented foods of different tribals of Manipur'. *Indian Journal of Traditional Knowledge*. 11: 70-77.

Dharshan, S., 2007. 'A future agenda for Indian medical heritage'. *Indian Anthropologist*. 37, 1: 173-186.

Grierson, GA., 1904. *Linguistic Survey of India*, Vol. III, Part III, Tibeto-Burman Family: Specimen of the Kuki-Chin and Burmese Group. Calcutta; Office of the Superintendent of Government Press.

Jain, SK., 2004. *A Manual of Ethnobotany*. Jodhpur; Scientific Publisher.

Kumar, GP., 2007. *Changing Healthcare Practicing among the Tribes*. pp. 308. Ambala Cantt. ; The Associated Publishers.

Kumari, P., 2006. 'Etiology and healing practices: A study in primitive societies of Jharkhand'. In P. Das Sharma (Ed): *Anthropology of Primitive Tribes in India*. pp. 487-499. New Delhi; Serial Publications.

Ray, A, and BV. Sharma, 2005. 'Ethnomedical beliefs and practices among the Savara'. In S. Sahay and PK. Singh (Eds): *Dimensions of Researchers in Indian Anthropology*, Volume II, pp. 454-464. New Delhi; Serials Publications.

Salehin, MA., 2012: '*Reproductive Health of Tribal Populations in India: A Sustainability Approach,* Unpublished Ph.D. thesis, The University of Texa at Arlington.

Sanglakpam, P., RR. Mathur and AK. Pandey, 2012. 'Ethnobotany of Chothe Tribe of Bishnupur District, Manipur'. *Indian Journal of Natural Products and Resources* 3: 414-425.

Chapter - 19

Indigenous Healthcare Systems: A Sumi Naga Perspective

—Kitoholi V. Zhimo

Introduction

The medical system of a society is inherently socio-cultural including not only systems of meanings and behavioural norms but also accompanying institutional settings and social relations (Kleinman, 1987). Healthcare systems, thus, articulate illness as a cultural idiom with a culturally specific, causation, symptomatizing illness behaviour, treatment, and alternatives, therapeutic practices etc., (*Ibid;* 86). The non-western societies, when viewed through such a lens, present a dynamic scenario of health, illness, and healthcare, where these are grounded in the cultural institutions and indigenous practices. As such, many authors (Simons, 1955; Suarez, 1974; Goode, 1962) attribute disease and illness among these societies to be variously influenced by sensate and/or on-sensate agent. Foster (1976), gave the two categories under which illnesses in most non-western society can be conveniently (not universally) placed – personalistic and naturalistic systems. In the personalistic system, the disease is explained as due to the "active purposeful intervention of an agent, who may be a human (a witch or sorcerer), non-human being (ghost, an ancestor or evil spirit) or supernatural being (a deity or other very powerful being). The sick person literally is a person, the object of aggression or punishment directed specifically against the same for certain reason concerned. Whereas, the naturalistic system explains illness's impersonal terms. Therefore, the disease is thought to stem, not from fear of an angry being but rather from such natural force or condition as cold, heat, wind, dampness and above all from an upset in the balance of the overall basic body elements.

The non-western societies of the North East India, thus, present an interesting scenario wherein not only the indigenous healthcare systems exhibit a wide array of knowledge and expertise but also face constant interactions with the increasingly infiltrating allopathic system of medicine and other forms of healthcare belonging to Indian systems of medicine. Thus, health and healthcare are understood and sought through increasingly overlapping sectors of healthcare, whereas the disease conception and terminology is largely based on native thought categories and cultural milieu, the causation, and therapeutic intervention often include professional sector like Allopathy and folk sectors of various spiritual and non-spiritual healers. Hence, one comes across a curious intermixing of different systems of healthcare leading to amalgamations of differently oriented health and healthcare practices depicting rich medical pluralism. So, where indigenous health system and practices still enjoy widespread of popular support and faith from the people of the Sumi tribe of Nagaland covering the folk and popular sector of healthcare, there exists a parallel plane where bio-medicine is fast becoming an accepted and demanding a choice of treatment. This chapter tries to present an overview of the indigenous healthcare and the embedded notion of illness, health, and disease. Following this, it attempts at locating various parallel functional medical system especially those of folk healing and biomedicine in contemporary times among the Sumi community of Nagaland. Thus, the objective of the present study is to understand the Indigenous healthcare system and related aspects and to analyse the interactions between the indigenous system and other professional systems of healthcare.

Universe of study

Nagaland is home to many tribal communities, of which Sumi community is counted as one of the major Naga tribes. Though dispersed in many areas of North East India, the Sumi community dominantly inhabits Dimapur and Zunheboto district of Nagaland. The Sumis have a rich history and cultural heritage around which they have spun an intricate web of social institutions and relations including a culturally relevant health system. With the advent of Christianity, this medical system of Sumi community has incorporated various facets in the personalistic domain of diseases. Another dimension in this regard is modern education which has introduced this community to the biomedical concept and other Indian healthcare systems of disease and treatment. Thus, the healthcare in present times exhibits a pluralistic scene where various health practices exist with each other and are adhered to variously by the Sumi community based on their discretion regarding the malady.

The data for the present chapter has been collected from the Sumi inhabiting the town of Satakha under Zunheboto District; however, some data has also been collected from a distance through informal consultations with other Sumi informants.

Methodology

The data collected for the present work employed a qualitative research frame including semi-structured interviews, key informant interviews, oral history, and telephonic conversations. The sample was purposively chosen and consisted of locals, folk healers, persons etc (both male and female) seeking treatment from both indigenous and biomedical systems and also sometimes from other Indian medical systems.

Being a native of universe studied, the problems of language and contextual significance of the data were mitigated. However, the effort was taken not to overlook the Sumi's notions and aspects in healthcare systems considered natural by us. Hence, the methodological rigor brings out an 'emic' perspective of the Sumi medical system.

For the analysis of the data collected, content analysis has been used through identifying themes and sub-themes.

Sumi Concept of Body, Health, Illness

To a Sumi, health is the state of being physically and mentally fit enough in such a manner that a person can maintain active and productive lifestyles in the day-to-day activities. This calls for the absence of any infirmity and weakness in the individual. The ethno physiology conception of the body is that of a machine that operates on power derived from consumption of food as a fuel. Various parts of the body with their associated organs function in accordance with each other in a circuit like a system. As such, the illness can be described in terms of impair functioning of some organ (s) or associated malfunction in any of the component as well as the accumulation of unwanted materials which hamper the normal smooth functioning of the organs in the body so here the impairment of function of the body organs may have both naturalistic and personalistic origin, the accumulation of unproductive materials (can be taken as dirt largely occurs due to personalistic forces). The ulterior aim in any of the aforementioned condition is always the restoring of the body parts and other organs to the normal active state. Both the folk healers as well as a biomedical therapist are expected to add in restoring the normal machinery functioning of the body in an episode of any illness. This explains the frequent jumping off by the Sumis from one system to another in order to seek an effective cure. This is again validated by the use of certain terminologies among the Sumis like herbalist might recommend a concoction 'to cleanse the stomach', a spiritual healer might pray 'may God wash out the dirt' in episodes of illnesses etc. Therefore, the Sumis combines the mechanical and plumbing model to explain body functioning and processes.

The Indigenous Healthcare Systems

In the present study, attempt is made to investigate indigenous healthcare systems in its totality of the universe of study enclosed and therefore have emphasised on the personalistic and naturalistic aspects of the same under which the folk and popular sector of both the domain is taken into account to comprehend the illness behaviour, causation, and treatment etc. The naturalistic etiological domain gets intermixed with the personalistic domain; however, it has been attempted to delimit both the domain for a clear understanding of which is presented in the further section.

Healthcare System Pertaining to Personalistic Etiology

The personalistic etiological domain of illness has an in-diminishable presence in the life of the Sumi community. One would find numerous instances when persons who otherwise attribute a disease to naturalistic causation, seek personalistic intervention for the pacification of that malady. This brings the picture of strong beliefs in religion and religious healers. Even though the pre-Christian animistic beliefs related to illness and associated magic have diminished following the advent of Christianity (Zhimo, 2011), the personalistic etiology among the Sumi have taken on a new shape by being incorporated into the institutions of the church. In this respect, "illness condition is brought about by the disharmony of vital powers that cause illness" (Kale, 1995). So, one comes across a multitude of folk healers variously known as prayer warriors, spiritual healers, priest, faith healers etc. They are held in high esteem and recognition, "traditional healers are enshrined in the minds of the people and respected in their community and they are often its opinion leaders" (*ibid,* 1995).

Those illness beliefs stemming from personalistic causes as such spirit intrusion, demon possessed, loss of spirit/soul, unstable condition under the influence of witchcraft or sorcery, etc. usually take up the form of extreme emotional behaviours like crying, uncontrollable aggressiveness, screaming, shouting, inflicting oneself with physical pain, bodily discomforts, mood disorder, unstable frame of mind etc., according to native's beliefs. In the preliminary stages, they seek measures of the popular sector for illness mitigation as the nearest available option that includes family members who come together in prayer, prayer warriors in the colony, or neighbours who are considered to be strong spiritually. Hereafter, in those cases where the illness is not mitigated and the condition of the victimized person becomes severe, the help from the socially recognised folk sector are sought in the form of spiritual healers recognised over a wider group within and outside the community, exorcist, priest, spiritist, etc. Some of this illness condition culturally considered to be caused in personalistic domain includes; *mhzamzha, tu-uli, alosukusu, tughu*

- *Mhzamhza* (loss of spirit/soul): A person is considered to have lost his spirit/soul which is taken away by the spirit locally known as *Mhzamhza*. This usually is thought to occur when the victim strays away in the thick jungles, crying in the forest, or calling out names loudly in the forest, etc. the spirit of that person in such a situation is sometimes thought to be trapped in the forest or encaged by the spirit. Also, *Mhzamhza* entices the person to lost track of his path by insisting it is a plane where it is the slope and run down the slope dragging the enticed person, slope where it is a plane and climbs up the slope slowly. The affected person suffers from loss of presence of mind, unstable mental condition, emotional disturbances, loss of appetite, inflicts physical harms in some case etc. This illness condition occurs irrespective of age and gender.
- *Tu-uli* (visitation of the dead in dream, sleep etc.): Here, the victim is said to be visited by the dead who had been his/her close acquaintance e.g. family members, relatives, neighbours, close friends, dead ancestors etc. with some intention of the visit such as unfulfilled wishes or whims, to taunt his/her enemy, to pacify loved ones, to torment the living if he/she is thought to die before his/her stipulated time such as in some accidents and tragedy etc. Therefore, the visitation is not always a harmful one. Here, the victim usually undergoes a period of a dilemma, emotional disturbances, psychological conflicts, anxiety, bafflement and more. To arrive at a positive outcome, prayer help is sought from prayer warriors, oracles, visions, etc. who communicates the underlying realities and the possible remedies to enhanced the victim back to normal condition. This illness condition also occurs irrespective of age and gender but usually, it is thought to occur in those people who were closely attached

to the deceased e.g. family members, close friends, a lover, or an enemy etc with some ulterior motives.

- *Alosukusu* (illness afflicted by Curse): Here, the illness is considered to be caused due to curse inflicted on the victim by ancestors who may be both dead and living due to certain reasons like disputes over property, rights, ill-treatment, and dissatisfaction over the victim's behaviours and role etc. The kinds of the curse that are known to be common and encountered among the natives are "may you never find happiness in life", "may you suffer like hell" and, "may you have no progenies". This usually results due to grievances and grudges that are nurtured over some unhappiness which brings about misfortunes and miseries to the victim and may occur irrespective of age and gender. The victim may suffer from natural calamities, misfortunes, poor health, no progeny etc. Besides, it is interesting to know even some disease conditions under naturalistic domain are also sometimes attributed to being caused by the same.
- *Tughu* (illness afflicted by poison/charms/ spell etc.): Although the history of Sumi community negates the practice of sorcery and witchcraft, some illness is believed to stem from the same, not from the native community but inflicted by people usually from other community, background etc. who are thought to involved in these practices. *Tughu* is a local term of Sumi which means poison and it is believed that the poison is hideously given to the victim mixed in food, water or the poison is inflicted through other means like doing witchcraft etc using the hair, clothes, materials etc of the victim. This occurs on grounds for several reasons such as jealousy, love charm, hatred, aggression etc. The affected person may lose inhibition of his own self, psychological disturbances, unstable mental condition, loss of appetite, depression, anxiety, aggressiveness, etc., thereby responding to the poison so inflicted. This illness condition can be afflicted to any person irrespective of age and gender against whom the grievances are nurtured.
- Satan/devil possessed: Here, the unstable condition that arises may be attributed to the intrusion of evil spirits in the body of the person due to various factors. The intruded person undergoes trance, psychological conflicts, and emotional disturbances, inflicts physical harm on oneself, loss of presence of mind, bodily disfigures, posed threats to the life of others attending to

him, etc. It is locally believed that those people who are weak spiritually and mentally are most likely to be possessed as such they appear as vulnerable victim to evil spirits. Possession of evil spirits is thought to occur irrespective of age and gender.

The curative measures for the mitigation for the above-mentioned illness condition, therefore, consult both the popular sector and folk sector according to the severity of the condition. Usually these spiritual healers cured the victims of spirit intrusion, demon possessed, loss of spirit/soul, unstable condition under the influence of witchcraft or sorcery etc. but frequently it happens that they are also consulted, either solely or simultaneously with other medicine to treat diseases like cancer, leprosy, inconceivable pregnancies and other medical condition which people themselves know and attributes to naturalistic cause. Moreover, one cannot overlook the fact according to the natives that, this invasion or the intrusion of the evil eye, supernatural power, curse etc. may sometimes also result in many other unpleasant medical conditions and therefore may seek the intervention of the same.

The spiritual healers in some case play a dual role in which besides giving spiritual healing and comforts from the disease and illness conditions, also administered the use of allopathic and other medical systems.

Types of Healers in Personalistic Domain

Spiritual healers: They could be male and female believed to have acquired the gift of vision, speaking in a tongue (communication with God), the power of healing from God and are considered as servants of God. They are sometimes considered equivalent to God who had attained spiritual powers of healing by the call of God. They have well recognised social roles in the society and are placed with utmost respect and dedication. Utilising the spiritual power gifted by God, these healers help in mitigating the disease causation attributed by various forces through prayer, vision etc. Some of the highly powerful spiritual healers are believed to have cured the patients not only illness caused by personalistic factors but also those diseases which are sometimes not cured by biomedicines and other medical systems such as cancer, leprosy etc. These powerful healers are thought to determine through vision as such the causes and nature of the illness by simply praying to God and at the same time avails healings for the same.

Prayer Warrior (s): This could be in a group or alone. They have less social roles than the spiritual healer and therefore sometimes could also be placed under popular sector. They also perform almost the same function as the spiritual healers although there may be some differences in the functions they perform according to the spiritual power they attained though the distinction is not to be argued. They perform the functions of driving out evil or Satan from the body of the person possessed, for loss of spirit, visitations of the dead, disturbances caused by the spirits etc. besides praying for other medical conditions rooted not only in personalistic but also very much in naturalistic origin.

Priests: They have well recognised social roles and responsibilities in the society and receive enormous respect and appraisal from the people. Every church has its own priest and therefore they attend to the needs of the people in the locality in the form of prayer support, consolation, moral support etc. They also cater to various aspects of praying and healing to the one in need. Not all priests obtain spiritual gifts of healing and vision but only those who had to attain higher call of pious life.

Exorcists: This includes prayer warriors, spiritual healers etc who take an active part in the personalistic intervention of illness and disease. They are believed to be very powerful and considered to deal especially with an evil spirit, demon, ghost etc which is thought to have entered the body of a person. They chased out the mentioned agents from the body by performing small rituals of reading Bible, prayer, touching the person with cross etc.

As mentioned earlier, these healers adhere not only to the personalistic orientation of disease causation and treatment but also are believed to have a significant role in mitigation of the disease in naturalistic as well as other biomedical orientation.

Healthcare Pertaining to Naturalistic Etiology

The naturalistic etiological domain covers the native categories of illness and disease intervention in both the popular sector and the folk sector as given in tables. The naturalistic domain which explains illness in impersonal term caters to the causative, illness behaviour and kind of treatment sought in both the sector. The disease intervention overlaps in both the sector but the treatment seek from this sector is oriented according to the native conception of severity and convenient. The native categories of disease and illness were comprehended in both the sectors according to their behavioural seeking for treatment and curative measures were undertaken. Whenever there is a situation of disease, the natives utilises the available curative measures of the popular sector as the first contact of self-medication. The disease and illness condition as such cold, fever, cough, gastric, headache, sinus, measles, migrant, piles, menstrual disorder, malaria, dysentery, cramps, body ache, cuts and wounds, boils, allergy of various kind as such wind, water, insect, food etc., insect bites, vomiting due to headache, fever etc., sore throat, natural births etc. The treatment for the mentioned disease and illness intervention in the form of self-help and self-medication are gained through consulting a person who is familiar with the condition such as doctor's wife, family members, women who are well verse and experience with child birth assisting for the same, ointments known popularly for some particular treatment such as *Moov, Vicks tablets, Disprin, Paracetamol, Digene, Safi, Chawanprash, Vicco Turmeric* etc.

Those diseases which are usually treated under popular sector may also be sought for treatment in the folk sector like fever, headache, sinus, pneumonia, jaundice, appendix, piles, ulcers etc. However, there are worse conditions which are considered indigenous to the Sumi community and which are consulted and healed by folk healers such as midwives, bone settlers, herbalist, and local massager etc. who may be both male and female. This illness in local term includes; *Asache, Annuhkusu, Azuamulukusu, Amlakusu, Apolalku, Aghisupsivekeu,* etc.

Table 19.1: Disease and illness conditions covering indigenous healthcare system

Domain	***Popular sector***	***Folk sector***	***Seeking behavior and treatment***
Persona-listic	Spirit intrusion, Satan possessed loss of spirit, visitation of the dead in sleep, dreams etc., illness condition due to curse by ancestors both living and dead etc.	Here, the illness intervention is some of the popular sectors. However, the orientation of illness may be glanced differently according to the severity and condition.	The first source of self-medication utilises popular sector and may include prayer supports from family members, relatives, neighbours, prayer warriors in the neighbourhood etc.In the folk sector, the mitigating measures for illness condition are sought from spiritual healers, prayer warriors, exorcist, priest etc.
Natura-listic	Cold, fever, headache, jaundice, appendix, pneumonia, sinus, measles, piles, dysentery, menstrual disorder, cough, sore throat, allergies....etc.	Those illness conditions in popular sector overlap in the folk sector in terms of curative measures and behaviours. *Asache, Azu Amuluh-kusu, Annuhkusu, Amlakusu, Apolaiku, Aghisupsikeu* etc.	The act of self-medication in the popular sector is gained through doctor's wife, family member recommending tablets or ointments for a particular illness, midwives, also self-utilisation of popular medicines like safi, disprin, paracetamol, Vicks tablets etc. The illness intervention in folk sector utilises the healing

(Cont'd...)

		These disease conditions are indigenous to the native.	consolation from bone settlers, local massagers, herbalists etc. Besides, folk healers also heal persons from several disease conditions mentioned in the popular sector.

The Table does not include an exhaustive list of disease and illness conditions in the universe under study. The maladies mentioned are indicative only.

Table 19.2: Native thought categories of naturalistic causation, behaviour and treatment

General Categories of illness	***Do's***	***Don't***
Sinus	Hot water steaming, intake water through the nose and vomit it through the mouth to cleanse and relief, warm food and water, soups etc.	Avoid cold food and water, limit unwanted exposure to cold air etc.
Pregnancy	Light exercise, i.e. walking, sweeping, etc after five months, from six months till delivery pregnant mother is encouraged to drink sugar cane juice to avoid jaundice in baby, intake of soups and meat of dog, chicken, crab, pigeon etc., as a source of medicinal supplements for the mother and the growing foetus.	Heavy exercise to be avoided, avoid crossing of shed-off skin of snake else it is believed that the baby so born acquires a skin like that of snake, a pregnant mother should not kill wild animals especially snake as when it is killed the baby born develops a hyperactive behavioural and restlessness, fruits like pineapple and papaya are thought to result in loss of foetus and so are avoided.
Jaundice	Intake sugarcane juice, sweet stuff etc. bark of mango tree is sliced and soaked and rubbed between the palms as curative measures against jaundice.	Avoid yellow stuff from food to clothing to other stuff, avoid intake of bitter stuff.
Appendix	Ingestion of boiled food, vegetables, soft and cooked food etc.	No roughage, avoid hard eatables such as betel nuts, avoid meat.
Piles	High intake of water, vegetables, use warm water for toilets, curative measures like putting heated salt in a cloth and placing it over the piles, soaked clothes in warm water and salt and repeats the same exercise, apply warm coconut oil to soften and soothe the piles.	Avoid intake of meat especially red meat.
Gastric	Intake gel of aloevera as a medicinal cure, less intake of spices, boiled vegetables, and food, lots of water.	Avoid spicy food, eat small meals at regular intervals, avoid staying up empty stomach, eat at regular timings.

Illness conditions indigenous to the locals and the causative, behavioural seeking, and treatment in folk sector are as follows:

Asache: This illness is considered as a condition when the blood clots in the head forming a spot where the hair becomes entangled and rough. As a result, the person suffers from a severe headache and develops feelings of vomiting. The folk healer expertise in this field usually heals the person suffering from this condition by systematically pulling out strands of hair wherever the spot is formed and massage the head. During this treatment, a snapping sound occurs and the clot is believed to be dissolved. Sometimes, the healers also make use of a mixture of crushed ginger and mustard oil and tie the same on the head of the person and leave the application for some duration. This doubles the relief of the pain. This illness condition has no age bar and therefore is widely common.

Annuhkusu: When a person suffers from this condition, the nervous system sometimes becomes impaired and a person cannot open or close the fist of the hand and toes, and other associated nervous dysfunctions occur in limbs or other body parts. This condition is healed by a folk healer by massaging systematically with mustard or any other oil for that matter in the body parts where the nerves are affected and brought back to its normalcy. This illness condition usually occurs in those people who have nerves problem and it can occur occasionally and/or in an unexpected situation too.

Azumuluhkusu: Here, the illness conditions are associated with the wind, water, climatic changes etc. The person considered to be affected by these agents complains of a backache, knee cramps, body pain, headache, bowel dysfunction etc. The folk healers usually make use of strongly scented plants, flowers, spices etc. such as marigold flower, ginger, and some other perfume and medicinal plants in native conception which are believed to keep these illness conditions under control and protect against the incoming forces with its scents. Besides these, the folk healers also use mustard oil or any other massaging oils, balm etc. to massage the affected area. The folk healer in this light is comparable to herbalists who make extensive use of medicinal plants and herbs etc. as they employed the same ideas of the herbalists in their treatment from the information obtained through social networks and relationships. This illness conditions can occur in every age group of both male and female but are usually common in middle-aged, old age, and those who are easily prone and sensitive to the changing weather conditions etc.

Amlakusu: This is an illness condition of the chest when a person develops a severe chest pain and suffers from a cough and cold. This illness condition in native terms can be associated with pneumonia as their symptoms are almost the same in their occurrence. It mostly occurs in a newborn baby, children, young people and old aged in minimum etc. This illness is considered to cause because of exposure to cold, wind, water etc. Some medicinal plants and herbs are given to the affected person beside massaging the same with warm oil, balm etc. by the folk healer and are advised to keep the body warm especially the chest, throat, feet etc.

Apolalku: In this illness condition the affected person is thought to be suffering from a dislocation of the umbilical cord of the navel which is anatomically located. This cause extreme pain and discomfort in the person as the cord is considered to be twisted inside. The folk healer checks the patient by taking a stick and placing it on the navel and lean it against the left side of the breast and repeat the exercise on the right side (or vice versa). It is said that if the stick does not meet the same measurement then there the dislocation of the cord is confirmed and the folk healer heals it by systematically massaging the affected area with oil. The affected person is also thought to be slapped against his/her heels simultaneously to bring the condition to normalcy. This illness can also occur in every age group.

Aghi Supsivekeu: This is a condition when the person suffers from the dislocation of the bones and sometimes nerves and muscles. It frequently occurs in newborn babies when the bone is not well developed and also among adults attributed by means of accident, fractures etc. The folk healers promote healing by locating the bone and massaging it with oil. They are thought to have knowledge of the entire body physical makeup and orientation.

As discussed previously, there are some disease conditions which are biological in origin but cater to curative measures in the folk sector. It is also interesting to note that although the causative nature of some diseases lies in the naturalistic domain according to native's etiology of disease causation, the curative measures are sought in the personalistic domain of healthcare. The underlying idea is that the strong faith and beliefs in the supreme power of the God deliver healings from every illness and disease.

Biomedicine, Pluralism and the Emerging Healthcare System

With the coming of new growth and development at the expense of globalisation, new healthcare systems have penetrated the core region of Nagaland. The rapid advancement in the era of modern science and technology contributes tremendously to the healthcare in the state. The forces of Western medicine and other Indian medical systems of healthcare cater to the eradication of various health problems which was once deemed impossible to get treated. Although there may be some kind of inadequacies in the medical systems in the remote corner of the state, yet following the increasing living standard of the people in towns and cities, the local people in the villages also cater to the incoming healthcare systems. The major health problems were collected in the desired universe by taking in account the native categories of diseases in a different orientation such as lifestyle disease, general disease, preventable disease, age onset disease etc. The common and major health illness that cater to biomedical treatment and other Indian medical systems includes diarrheal diseases, parasitic infection, infective hepatitis, enteric fever, water-borne diseases, piles, anaemia, respiratory disease, malaria, alcohol-related morbidity and conditions, IV drugs, HIV specifically MCH, tuberculosis, leprosy, asthma, jaundice, pneumonia, dysentery, sinus, appendix, measles, lungs cancer, kidney failure, liver malfunctioning, cancer of various kinds such as throat, mouth, blood, brain etc. The biomedical systems and those of Indian medical systems adhere for the mitigation of listed diseases and health problems.

The advancement in modern medicine and other Indian medical systems (ISM), do not diminish the traditional systems and practice of medicine rooted in the indigenous identity of the local people. These traditional systems of medicine can be in the form of the folk identity of spiritual healing, herbalists, bone setters, midwives, prayer warriors, and several other types of folk healers etc. and some firsthand treatment of self-medication covering the naturalistic etiology. As a result, there is a kind of coexistence of modern medicine and the indigenous healthcare systems which give an interesting picture of the universe studied. In the present study, an attempt has been made to explore the how indigenous system interacts with other medical system and how this goes hand in hand. There remains a parallel plane where indigenous health systems travel in continuity with other medical systems. "Some patients see traditional healers exclusively, but many others see their healer before, during or after treatment by a modern doctor" (Kale, 1995). The present scenario of Sumi community (specific to area studied), reflects a dualistic nature of health systems where their indigenous systems interact and exists with other medical systems. For example; in the earlier times, people preferred a large family with most families having more than five children sometimes amounting to 10 to 13 or more. The delivery of all these birth was natural in the absence of high-tech caesarean operation. The discouraging fact is the complication that arises out of the complexities of health in the modern era of science and technology that people are encouraged to adopt operative measures of delivery rather than natural birth. Therefore, with the development of healthcare sectors especially in the field of biomedicine and its related treatment, there is a significant decrease of childbirth through natural delivery systems. But this has not left behind the traditional system of child delivery by midwives, a woman who is experienced in this field etc. and it still operates in those regions where the proper medical arrangement has not reach and also accessed by people who are economically weak. This throws a light on how the traditional system still exists in continuity with the growing healthcare systems. Besides, various folk healers still serve to mitigate the illness and disease conditions in line with the biomedicine and other Indian systems of medicine such as Ayurveda, homeopathy, acupressure etc. There is also disease and illness conditions where people seek the intervention of the existing source of treatment of more than one. As such, in some cases, a person suffering from a medical condition and seeking medical treatment for the same, may also seek to heal from the folk healers such as spiritual healer. The firm believes in the supreme power of God hold a prominent place in a strong believer of Christianity and it culminates to their illness seeking behaviour which they believed will diminish the unease condition of the body and related problems. Therefore, a believer in Christ may seek treatment from the modern medicine but at the same time, the faiths in his religion provoke him to seek to heal from spiritual healers, prayers, etc. In such situation, when the person successful comes out of some operations, treatments etc. the gratitude is paid to God for the people believe that mission is accomplished through Him. It is also natively believed that some complicated medical condition such as cancer, leprosy etc. when to bring into the personalistic domain, is treated and mitigated by the healing power obtained from the folk healers utilising supernatural origin. Some of these spiritual healers even prescribed the patients to utilise allopathic medicines in some disease condition beside the consolation healing that are given which contributes to the amalgamations of one or more medical systems. This brings about the emergence of the new medical systems wherein the roots of folk healing and tradition are incorporated into the newly increasing biomedicines, "Western biomedicines and Indigenous traditional healthcare systems have different concepts and practices and run in parallel, sometimes together and sometimes in opposition" (Laura and Bishop, 2000).

Table 19.3: Native categories of disease under different orientation seeking biomedical treatment

Native categories of disease conditions			
General	***Lifestyles***	***Preventable***	***Age onset***
Sinus, piles, appendix, intestinal problems, diabetics*, jaundice, gastric, menstrual disorders, migraine, infections, body cramps ….etc.	Liver and kidney failure (due to alcohol), lungs cancer (smoking cigarettes, weeds etc.), malaria (unhygienic environment that allows mosquitoes breeding etc), polio, small pox, chicken pox (due to no timely vaccine), diabetics, mouth and throat cancer (due to chewing tobaccos etc), HIV and AIDS (drugs, unprotected sex or multiple sexual partners, unsterilised needles etc.)	Malaria, dysentery, polio*, small pox*, Chicken pox*, pneumonia, typhoid, water and airborne disease (living in unhygienic conditions), malaria*, HIV and AIDS*,	Cataract, impaired vision and hearing, blood pressure, cardiac arrest, arthritis, osteoarthritis, heart problems, osteoporosis, diabetes etc.

* Some disease conditions overlap in the given categories.

Discussions

This chapter focus on the indigenous health systems and their behaviour of seeking treatment, which in the present study uncover that people adhere to self-medication, folk healing etc. without or in isolation with modern science depending on the severity of the conditions, as a result enhancing changing the treatment seeking behaviour according to the availability of the same; it does not diminish the existence but other health systems (Niraula, 1994). Traditional healers are an integral part of the people and society; they are inborn in it, they know the way of the people and work for the good of the people and also complement the modern medical systems, for example, Prof Kirsch (cited in Kale, 1995) gave an account of one of his patient with a psychological problem in his ward, who did not respond to modern medical treatment but bringing him in contact with the traditional healer, the patient condition improved in one session. (*ibid*, 1995). The attempt in the chapter to explore the pluralistic nature of indigenous systems with other medical systems lay in line with many scholars, "traditional medical systems co-exist and complement western scientific or modern medicine" (Goode, 1997).The interaction between indigenous and modern science is increasing, they complement or work in unison, "Physicians in some non-Western societies, such as even in India, work alongside practitioners of traditional medical systems" (Jingfing, 1987 cited in Linda, 1995). The same has been echoed by many scholars; Offering, 1999; Caoromaero and Bishop, 2000 as such all this situation of modern medical and traditional systems continues to generate a debate as to whether these two systems can ever be integrated or not? (Offioing, 1999). WHO as an organisation has established a new department; "The Traditional Medicine Programme" that urges the member's states to integrate indigenous healers into the general health systems. (Jingfing, 1987 cited in Linda, 1995).In the present chapter, an attempt has been made to look into the emergence of the new medical system incorporated by the traditional system with biomedical and other healthcare systems of India. Integration or not, traditional systems remain the very embodiment of the conscience of the societies (Offioing, 1999), and continue to engage in pluralistic orientation which has become accepted elsewhere, "Medical pluralism, the co-existence and the use of various forms of modern and traditional medical system, is a well-recognised phenomenon in many developed countries" (Phillips, 1992).

Conclusion

Not much work has been done among the tribes of North East India regarding healthcare and associated systems of therapy. Therefore, systematic inquiries into the conception of health, healthcare and the associated nosologies and the whole systems of healing and cure make a focus area for research. The indigenous system of healing among Sumi Community has to be thoroughly comprehended in order to better understand and look for future implications in the choice, rationale, and associated behaviour for seeking healthcare by the Sumis as there has been a complex intermixing of the folk systems of healing with the biomedical system of medicines and neither has replaced or subsided any one system. In addition, another point that emerges from the analysis is that unlike the mainland tribes which have been in close association with the Indian medical system thereby internalising those systems into folk domain of healing; the Sumi community subscribe to somewhat different kind of medical system wherein the professional sector of ISM is as much a newer introduction to the pre-existing Sumi health system as is the biomedical systems. This in turns complex the interaction of various systems, giving more options to thc Sumis on one hand and calling for a rectification in the already existing thought categories of Sumis. This study acts as a small attempt in order to understand the pluralistic nature of healthcare and the place of the indigenous system in healthcare behaviour of the Sumis. However, further studies are needed to fully understand, evaluate and arrive at the dynamics of complex interactions of the various systems and how these can be fully utilised for an effective in the Sumi society.

References

Anyinam, Charles, 1987. 'Availability, accessibility, acceptability, and adaptability: Four attributes of African ethnomedicine'. *Social Science and Medicine*. 25, 7: 803-811.

Foster, GM, and BG. Anderson, 1987. *Medical Anthropology*. New York; Wiley.

Foster, GM., 1976. 'Disease etiologies in non-western medical systems'. *American Anthropologist*, 78, 4: 773-782.

Goode, BG., 1977. 'The heart of what's the matter: The semantics of illness in Iran'. *Culture, Medicine, and Psychiatry*, 1: 25-58.

Goode, CM., 1997. 'Traditional Medicine: An agenda for medical geography'. *Social Science and Medicine*, 11: 705-713.

Hardiman, D, and Gauri Raje. 2008. 'Practices of healing in tribal Gujarat'. *Economic and Political Weekly*, 43, 9: 43-50.

Kale, Rajendra, 1995. 'Traditional healers in South Africa: A parallel healthcare system'. *British Medical Journal*. 6988, 310:1182-1185.

Kleinman, A., 1978. 'Concepts and a model for the comparison of medical systems as cultural systems'. *Social Science and Medicine*, 12:83-93.

Laura Caoromaero and Alina Bishop, 2000. 'Don't forget traditional medical care'. *British Medical Journal*. 321, 7264: 831-832.

Leslie, C., 1976. *Introduction to Asian Medical Systems*: *A Comparative Study*. Berkley; University of California Press.

Linda Blerkom, MV. 1995. 'Clown doctors: Shaman healers of western medicine'. *Medical Anthropology*. 9, 4:462-475.

Madan, TN., 1969. 'Who chooses modern medicine and why'. *Economic and Political Weekly*, 4, 37: 1475-1484.

Niraula, BB., 1994. 'Use of health services in hill villages in Central Nepal'. *Health Transition Review*, 4, 2: 151-166.

Offiong, DA., 1999. 'Traditional healers in the Nigerian healthcare delivery system and the debate over integrating traditional and scientific'. *Anthropologist Quarterly*, 72, 3: 118-130.

Paul, BK., 1985. 'Approaches to medical geography: A historical perspective'. *Social Science and Medicine*, 20, 4: 399-409.

Philips, DR., 1992. 'A comparison of the use of traditional and modern medicine in primary health centres in Tamil Naidu'. *Geo Journal*, 26, 1: 21-30.

Zhimo, AV., 2011. 'Culture, identity, and change: The case of the Sumi of Nagaland'. *Indian Anthropologist*, 41, 2: 33-48.

Index

W